Natural Healing Handbook

Essential herbal Remedies to Restore Your Body's Ability to Heal Itself, Boost Immunity, Promote Wellness, and Enhance Your Well-Being

Ruby Kenyon

Table of contents

Chapter 1 5
    Understanding the Body's Healing Power 5
    The Concept of Holistic Health and Healing 5
    The Mind-Body Connection 7
    Why Natural Healing Works 9
    The Role of the Immune System in Healing and Disease Prevention 13

Chapter 2 17
    Preparing Your Body for Healing 17
    The Importance of a Balanced Diet in Maintaining Wellness 20

Chapter 3 30
    Immunity Boosters 30

Chapter 4 42
    Respiratory Health 42

Chapter 5 54
    Digestive Health 54

Chapter 6 67
    Skin Health and Healing 67
    Lavender Oil: Soothing for Burns, Acne, and Skin Infections 73

Chapter 7 79
    Pain and Inflammation Relief 79

Chapter 8 91

- Mental Wellness and Stress Relief 91

Chapter 9 103

- The Role of Mindfulness in Healing 103
- Practicing Meditation for Stress Relief and Emotional Healing 104
- Deep Breathing Exercises to Activate the Parasympathetic Nervous System 107
- Visualization Techniques for Healing and Overcoming Mental Barriers 111

Chapter 10 116

- Restorative Practices for the Body and Spirit 116
- The Power of Yoga and Stretching for Physical and Mental Rejuvenation 117
- Essential Oils for Relaxation and Spiritual Grounding 121
- The Importance of Nature and Outdoor Activities in Holistic Health 125

Chapter 11 129

- Creating a Healing Space 129
- How to Design a Nurturing Environment for Rest and Recovery 130
- The Benefits of Natural Elements 134
- Incorporating Healing Herbs and Remedies into Your Daily Routine 137
- Building a Natural Medicine Cabinet 142

Chapter 12 145

- Prevention through Natural Healing 145

Maintaining Long-Term Health and Wellness..........145

Building a Routine to Prevent Common Ailments and Chronic Diseases 146

The Importance of Regular Herbal Detoxes and Cleanses 151

Chapter 13 158

Embracing the Future of Natural Healing 158

Building a Sustainable, Holistic Lifestyle for Long-Term Health 161

Chapter 1

Understanding the Body's Healing Power

The body is an extraordinary and complex system, designed to heal itself when given the right tools and conditions. In modern society, we often turn to medications and treatments to address physical ailments, but for centuries, people have turned to natural remedies to promote wellness and restore balance. This chapter delves into the foundational principles of natural healing, providing an understanding of the power that resides within each of us to heal, rejuvenate, and maintain good health through natural methods.

The Concept of Holistic Health and Healing

Holistic health is an approach that considers the whole person—mind, body, and spirit—in the pursuit of wellness. The term "holistic" comes from the word "whole," emphasizing the interconnectedness of various aspects of our being. Unlike traditional medicine, which often isolates symptoms and treats them independently, holistic health views the body as a complex system where physical, mental, emotional, and spiritual health are deeply interwoven. A person cannot be truly healthy if one aspect of their being is neglected or out of balance.

In holistic health, the focus is on restoring balance and harmony within the body and mind, with the understanding that everything from our thoughts and emotions to our diet and lifestyle choices affects our overall health. Healing, therefore, is not just about treating disease, but about nurturing the body, mind, and spirit to work together harmoniously. This is why natural healing methods—such as the use of herbs, diet, meditation, and exercise—are central to holistic health practices.

Natural healing taps into the body's inherent ability to regenerate and restore balance, using gentle, non-invasive techniques that promote self-healing without the need for synthetic medications or aggressive interventions. Whether it's through nutrition, herbal remedies, or mindful practices, holistic healing empowers individuals to become active participants in their health journey.

The Mind-Body Connection

One of the most profound aspects of holistic health is the mind-body connection. The emotional and psychological states we experience have a direct impact on our physical health. This connection is well-documented in scientific research, with studies showing that chronic stress, negative emotions, and unresolved psychological issues can manifest in physical symptoms such as headaches, digestive problems, high blood pressure, and even chronic illnesses like heart disease.

When we experience stress or negative emotions like anger, fear, or anxiety, our bodies respond by releasing stress hormones such as cortisol. In small doses, cortisol can be helpful, as it prepares the body for a "fight or flight" response. However, when stress is chronic, prolonged elevated cortisol levels can lead to various health problems, including weakened immune function, inflammation, and disruptions in metabolic processes. These physiological changes not only make the body more vulnerable to illness, but they also slow down the body's ability to heal itself.

On the other hand, positive emotions such as love, joy, and peace promote the release of beneficial hormones like oxytocin, serotonin, and endorphins, which have healing properties. These hormones can boost immune function, reduce inflammation, and improve overall well-being. Practices like mindfulness meditation, yoga, and deep breathing exercises have been shown to lower cortisol levels, reduce stress, and activate the body's natural healing processes.

Herbal medicine also acknowledges the connection between the mind and body, recognizing that the emotional state plays a significant role in physical health. Many herbs, such as chamomile, lavender, and ashwagandha, have calming properties that help reduce anxiety and stress, thereby promoting overall health. These herbs work not only on a physical level but also on an emotional level, helping to bring the body and mind into a state of balance.

Why Natural Healing Works

The healing properties of plants and natural substances have been well known for thousands of years. From the ancient civilizations of Egypt, China, and India, to modern-day herbalists and naturopaths, the use of herbs and natural remedies has stood the test of time. But why do these natural healing methods work?

The science behind herbal medicine lies in the chemical compounds that plants contain, many of which have been shown to have therapeutic effects on the body. These compounds interact with the body in various ways, supporting or enhancing physiological functions to bring about healing. For example, many herbs contain antioxidants that help to fight free radicals—unstable molecules that damage cells and contribute to aging and disease. Other herbs contain compounds that have anti-inflammatory, antimicrobial, or analgesic properties, which can help alleviate symptoms and promote healing.

Take, for example, the herb turmeric, which contains a compound called curcumin. Curcumin has been extensively studied for its powerful anti-inflammatory and antioxidant properties. It can help reduce pain and swelling in conditions like arthritis, and it has also been shown to support brain function, improve digestion, and fight cancer. Similarly, garlic contains allicin, a sulfur compound known for its antibacterial, antiviral, and antifungal properties. This makes garlic an excellent remedy for boosting the immune system, fighting infections, and promoting cardiovascular health.

Herbal remedies are often more gentle on the body than synthetic drugs because they work in harmony with the body's natural processes, rather than forcing the body into a specific state. For example, herbs like echinacea and elderberry work by stimulating the immune system, allowing the body to fight off infections more effectively. Unlike antibiotics, which can disrupt the delicate balance of bacteria in the gut and lead to resistance, these herbs support the body's own defense mechanisms, helping it to heal without causing long-term harm.

Additionally, many herbal remedies come with fewer side effects compared to prescription drugs, which often include harsh chemicals that can cause unwanted reactions. Natural remedies, in contrast, are typically gentler and more suited for long-term use. For instance, chamomile is often used as a calming tea to treat insomnia, anxiety, and digestive issues, and it is widely considered safe for long-term use without the risk of addiction or side effects that may be associated with pharmaceutical sedatives.

While herbal remedies have gained popularity in modern wellness culture, they are deeply rooted in traditional healing practices. The body's healing power is supported by natural ingredients that enhance its ability to restore balance, strengthen its defenses, and prevent disease.

The Role of the Immune System in Healing and Disease Prevention

At the heart of the body's ability to heal itself lies the immune system. The immune system is a complex network of cells, tissues, and organs that work together to defend the body against harmful invaders such as bacteria, viruses, fungi, and toxins. The immune system's primary role is to recognize and destroy pathogens before they can cause harm to the body. It is also responsible for identifying and eliminating damaged or infected cells, thus preventing diseases like cancer.

Natural healing methods, particularly herbs, play a significant role in supporting the immune system. Many herbs and natural remedies have immune-boosting properties that help to enhance the body's ability to fight infections and prevent illness. For example, echinacea is one of the most well-known herbs for immune support. It has been shown to increase the production of white blood cells, which are responsible for identifying and attacking harmful pathogens. Similarly, elderberry is rich in antioxidants and has been shown to prevent the replication of flu viruses, reducing the duration and severity of illness.

The immune system is also linked to the body's ability to recover from injury or illness. A strong immune response speeds up recovery time and helps to reduce the risk of complications. This is why maintaining a healthy immune system is essential for overall health and well-being. Natural remedies, including proper nutrition, adequate sleep, regular exercise, and stress management, all contribute to a robust immune system.

In addition to herbs, nutrition plays a crucial role in strengthening the immune system. Nutrient-rich foods, such as fruits and vegetables high in vitamin C (e.g., oranges, strawberries, and bell peppers), zinc (e.g., pumpkin seeds, legumes), and antioxidants (e.g., blueberries, spinach), help to fuel the body's immune response. A balanced diet rich in these nutrients ensures that the body has the necessary resources to fight off infections and recover from illness.

Natural healing not only supports the immune system but also teaches us the importance of prevention. By taking steps to nourish our bodies and minds, we can prevent disease before it starts. A lifestyle that prioritizes nutrition, stress management, and rest will naturally strengthen the immune system, helping to keep us healthy and resilient in the face of illness.

In conclusion, the body's healing power is a profound and intrinsic force, supported by natural remedies, the mind-body connection, and a holistic approach to health. By understanding how emotions and thoughts impact physical health, why natural remedies work, and the crucial role of the immune system, we can begin to embrace a lifestyle that promotes healing from within. Through the use of herbal remedies, mindful practices, and a balanced diet, we can unlock the body's full potential to restore itself to optimal health.

Chapter 2

Preparing Your Body for Healing

In the journey toward natural healing, the first step is preparing the body to restore balance and rejuvenate. Healing does not happen in isolation; it requires an environment that is clean, well-nourished, hydrated, and rested. This chapter explores four essential components of preparation: detoxification, a balanced diet, proper hydration, and quality sleep. These foundational elements support the body's healing process, laying the groundwork for a healthier and more vibrant you.

Detoxification: Why Cleansing Your Body is Essential for Health

Detoxification is the body's natural process of eliminating or neutralizing toxins through organs such as the liver, kidneys, and intestines. Toxins can come from a variety of sources, including the food we eat, the air we breathe, environmental pollutants, and even stress. Over time, if the body becomes overwhelmed with toxins, it can lead to a buildup that interferes with normal bodily functions, weakens the immune system, and impedes the healing process.

The purpose of detoxification is to support the body's ability to naturally cleanse itself of harmful substances, allowing it to restore balance and function optimally. Detoxification goes beyond just "flushing out" toxins; it is about supporting the body's natural ability to repair and regenerate. The liver, which is the body's primary detoxification organ, plays a pivotal role in processing and filtering out harmful substances. A healthy liver is critical for maintaining good health, as it helps to remove waste products and toxins from the bloodstream.

Several natural methods can help to support and enhance detoxification, including fasting, juicing, herbal teas, and eating nutrient-dense foods that support liver and kidney function. For instance, dandelion root is an herb known for its liver-detoxifying properties, promoting the removal of waste products and toxins. Similarly, milk thistle has been used for centuries to support liver function and protect it from damage caused by toxins.

One of the simplest and most effective ways to support detoxification is by consuming fresh fruits and vegetables that are rich in antioxidants, which help neutralize free radicals in the body. Foods like beets, cruciferous vegetables (like broccoli and cabbage), and garlic stimulate liver enzymes and help facilitate detoxification. Additionally, green tea is packed with antioxidants that help support the body's detox process, while herbs like ginger and turmeric possess anti-inflammatory properties that can assist in the removal of toxins from the body.

However, it is important to approach detoxification with care. While the body has its own natural detoxifying mechanisms, using herbs and juices should not be used as a quick fix but rather as part of a long-term, sustainable lifestyle that prioritizes healthy eating, hydration, and regular exercise. Regularly supporting detoxification through these natural practices helps to optimize the body's natural healing capabilities.

The Importance of a Balanced Diet in Maintaining Wellness

Nutrition is the foundation of health. Without a proper diet, the body cannot function properly, and healing becomes a much slower and more difficult process. A balanced diet ensures that the body receives the necessary vitamins, minerals, and nutrients required for optimal functioning. These nutrients not only fuel the body but also promote healing, strengthen the immune system, and support the body's ability to regenerate and repair itself.

A balanced diet includes a variety of whole, unprocessed foods from different food groups. The key to a truly balanced diet is variety—eating a wide range of colorful fruits and vegetables, healthy fats, lean proteins, and whole grains. Each food group provides essential nutrients that the body needs to thrive.

- Fruits and Vegetables: These are packed with essential vitamins, minerals, and antioxidants. For example, vitamin C-rich foods like oranges, strawberries, and bell peppers support immune function and collagen production, aiding in the healing of tissues. Leafy greens like spinach and kale provide magnesium, which plays a role in muscle function and relaxation. Additionally, the fiber in fruits and vegetables helps regulate digestion and supports the body's natural detoxification processes.

•	Healthy Fats: Healthy fats, particularly those from plant-based sources like avocados, nuts, and seeds, are essential for maintaining cellular health, reducing inflammation, and supporting the brain. Omega-3 fatty acids, found in foods such as chia seeds, flaxseeds, and fatty fish like salmon, are particularly beneficial for reducing inflammation, which is critical in the healing process.

•	Lean Proteins: Proteins are the building blocks of the body and play a vital role in the repair and regeneration of tissues. Consuming lean proteins such as chicken, turkey, and legumes helps provide amino acids necessary for tissue repair, muscle growth, and immune function. For vegetarians or vegans, tofu, lentils, and quinoa are excellent plant-based protein sources.

- Whole Grains: Whole grains like brown rice, quinoa, oats, and barley provide the body with complex carbohydrates that offer sustained energy, regulate blood sugar levels, and provide fiber for digestive health. Unlike refined grains, whole grains are rich in essential nutrients such as B vitamins, iron, and magnesium.

Alongside these food groups, a balanced diet also involves avoiding or minimizing processed foods that are high in sugar, refined carbohydrates, and unhealthy fats. These foods can cause inflammation, disrupt metabolic processes, and contribute to the development of chronic diseases, making it harder for the body to heal.

In addition to eating a variety of nutrient-dense foods, practicing mindful eating is just as important. Eating in a relaxed and focused manner helps improve digestion and nutrient absorption, giving the body the best chance to assimilate essential nutrients. By taking the time to nourish the body with healthy foods, we support the body's natural healing process and promote overall wellness.

Hydration: The Vital Role Water Plays in Natural Healing

Water is life, and hydration is the cornerstone of health and wellness. The human body is composed of approximately 60% water, and every cell, tissue, and organ in the body relies on water to function properly. When the body is adequately hydrated, all physiological processes, including detoxification, digestion, nutrient absorption, and circulation, can occur more efficiently.

Water is particularly important during the healing process because it helps to flush toxins from the body, lubricates joints, aids digestion, and facilitates nutrient transport to cells. When the body is dehydrated, these processes slow down, and the body becomes less efficient at healing and maintaining balance. Dehydration can also cause a wide range of symptoms, including fatigue, headaches, dry skin, and digestive problems, which can further hinder the body's ability to recover.

In addition to pure water, herbal teas and infused water with fruits and herbs also help support hydration and healing. For instance, lemon water is an excellent detoxifier, providing vitamin C and promoting liver function, while ginger tea aids digestion and reduces inflammation. Coconut water is another great option for replenishing electrolytes after exercise or illness, making it an ideal hydration source for recovery.

The recommended daily intake of water varies depending on factors such as age, activity level, and climate, but a general rule of thumb is to aim for at least eight 8-ounce glasses of water a day. It's important to listen to your body's thirst signals, as well, and hydrate more frequently if you're engaging in physical activity, experiencing hot weather, or undergoing illness or detoxification.

Adequate hydration helps the body function at its best, enabling the organs to perform their detoxification and regeneration functions and providing the necessary environment for healing.

Sleep: How Quality Rest Accelerates the Healing Process

Sleep is often overlooked in the modern world, but it is one of the most crucial elements of the healing process. During sleep, the body undergoes significant restorative processes, including tissue repair, immune system regeneration, and the consolidation of memories. Without sufficient sleep, the body struggles to heal and recover, leading to chronic fatigue, impaired immune function, and a weakened ability to manage stress.

When we sleep, the body produces growth hormone, which plays a vital role in tissue repair and cell regeneration. The immune system also becomes more active during sleep, working to fight off infections and diseases. Inadequate sleep can reduce the body's ability to fight infections, which in turn slows down the healing process. Sleep also allows the body to process emotions and relieve stress, contributing to mental and emotional well-being.

Quality sleep is just as important as quantity. Ensuring that sleep is uninterrupted and restorative is crucial for healing. Establishing a sleep routine, reducing exposure to blue light before bedtime, and creating a calm, relaxing environment can significantly improve sleep quality. Herbal remedies like lavender and chamomile tea can also promote relaxation and improve sleep quality.

Generally, adults need between 7-9 hours of sleep per night to function optimally, although this can vary. Paying attention to sleep hygiene, managing stress, and creating a sleep-friendly environment are key to ensuring that the body gets the rest it needs for healing.

In conclusion, preparing your body for healing involves more than just applying remedies—it requires nurturing the body through detoxification, a balanced diet, proper hydration, and quality sleep. By taking the time to support these essential areas, you provide the body with the foundation it needs to restore itself, recover from illness, and maintain long-term wellness. Natural healing begins with taking care of the body's basic needs and creating an environment conducive to optimal health.

Chapter 3

Immunity Boosters

The immune system is the body's first line of defense against illness, pathogens, and diseases. It is responsible for recognizing harmful invaders and mounting an appropriate response to neutralize them. A strong immune system is essential for health and well-being, as it helps to prevent infections, promote recovery, and maintain balance in the body. This chapter will explore four powerful natural remedies—echinacea, elderberry, ginger & turmeric, and garlic—that are known for their ability to boost immune function, fight infections, and support overall health.

Echinacea: The Powerhouse Herb for Fighting Infections and Boosting the Immune System

Echinacea, also known as purple coneflower, is one of the most widely used and researched herbs for immune support. This native North American plant has been used for centuries by indigenous peoples for its medicinal properties, particularly for treating infections, colds, and respiratory issues. Echinacea is often regarded as a "go-to" herb for boosting immune health, especially during cold and flu season.

The primary components in echinacea that contribute to its immune-boosting properties are alkamides, polysaccharides, and flavonoids. These compounds work synergistically to enhance the activity of white blood cells, which are responsible for fighting off infections. Echinacea has been shown to stimulate the production of cytokines, molecules that are essential for immune responses, and increase the activity of phagocytes, the cells that engulf and destroy pathogens.

Several studies have demonstrated that echinacea can reduce the duration and severity of cold symptoms. It is believed that echinacea works by stimulating the immune system, preventing the virus from proliferating, and supporting the body's natural defenses. Some research suggests that when taken at the onset of a cold or flu, echinacea can reduce symptoms by up to 50% and shorten the duration of illness.

Echinacea is most effective when used as a preventive measure or during the early stages of an illness. It can be taken in various forms, including tinctures, capsules, lozenges, or teas. While it is generally considered safe for short-term use, it's important to note that people with autoimmune conditions or allergies to the daisy family of plants (such as ragweed) should consult a healthcare provider before using echinacea.

Elderberry: A Potent Antiviral Remedy for Colds and Flu

Elderberry, derived from the Sambucus nigra plant, has long been used in traditional medicine as a remedy for respiratory infections, especially colds and flu. The small, dark berries of the elderberry plant are packed with antioxidants, vitamins, and bioflavonoids that support immune health and help to ward off infections. Elderberry is particularly known for its ability to act as a potent antiviral, helping to fight off viruses and prevent the spread of infection.

The key active compounds in elderberry are anthocyanins, a type of antioxidant that gives elderberries their dark color and provides many of their medicinal properties. Anthocyanins have been shown to inhibit the ability of viruses to enter human cells, thereby reducing the severity and duration of illnesses like the common cold and the flu. Elderberry has been shown to be effective against the influenza virus and may even shorten the duration of flu symptoms when taken within the first 48 hours of exposure.

In addition to its antiviral properties, elderberry is rich in vitamin C and flavonoids, both of which support the immune system and help to fight inflammation. Elderberry also contains compounds that have anti-inflammatory effects, which can alleviate symptoms like congestion, sinus pressure, and body aches associated with colds and flu.

Elderberry can be consumed in a variety of forms, including syrups, teas, lozenges, and capsules. It is particularly popular during the winter months when colds and flu are more prevalent, but it can be taken year-round to boost immunity. Elderberry is generally considered safe for most people; however, it is important to note that raw elderberries and other parts of the plant can be toxic, so they should never be consumed unless they are properly prepared, typically through cooking or processing into syrups.

Ginger & Turmeric: Anti-Inflammatory Herbs That Support Immunity and Overall Wellness

Ginger and turmeric are two powerful herbs that have been used for centuries in traditional medicine for their anti-inflammatory, immune-boosting, and overall wellness-promoting properties. Both of these herbs contain potent compounds that support immune health, reduce inflammation, and promote general well-being.

•	Ginger: Ginger, scientifically known as Zingiber officinale, is a well-known digestive aid and an anti-inflammatory powerhouse. The primary bioactive compound in ginger, gingerol, gives it its spicy flavor and contributes to its medicinal properties. Ginger has been shown to enhance immune function by stimulating the production of white blood cells, which are vital for fighting infections. It also has powerful antioxidant properties that help to combat oxidative stress and protect the body from free radical damage.

Ginger is also known for its ability to reduce inflammation in the body, which makes it particularly effective for conditions like arthritis, digestive issues, and respiratory problems. In addition to its immune-boosting and anti-inflammatory effects, ginger is commonly used to alleviate nausea, improve digestion, and support cardiovascular health.

Ginger can be consumed in a variety of ways, including ginger tea, fresh ginger root, ginger powder, or ginger supplements. Drinking ginger tea, especially during the colder months, is a soothing and effective way to support the immune system and promote general health.

- Turmeric: Turmeric, or Curcuma longa, is a yellow-orange root that has gained popularity worldwide due to its powerful anti-inflammatory and immune-boosting properties. The active compound in turmeric, curcumin, is responsible for many of its health benefits. Curcumin has been extensively studied for its ability to reduce inflammation, modulate immune responses, and support overall health.

Curcumin works by inhibiting the activity of pro-inflammatory enzymes and promoting the activity of anti-inflammatory cytokines in the body. This makes turmeric a potent herb for addressing chronic inflammation, which is associated with a wide range of health conditions, including autoimmune diseases, arthritis, and heart disease. Moreover, curcumin supports the immune system by promoting the production of T-cells, which play a critical role in defending the body against infections.

Turmeric is often used in traditional dishes such as curries and soups, and it can also be consumed as a tea or in supplement form. However, curcumin is poorly absorbed by the body on its own, so it is often paired with black pepper or healthy fats (such as coconut oil) to enhance absorption.

Both ginger and turmeric can be used together to provide a powerful combination of anti-inflammatory and immune-boosting effects. Whether taken as part of a warm, soothing tea or added to meals, these herbs offer a natural and effective way to support the body's defense systems.

Garlic: Nature's Antibiotic for Infections and Strengthening the Immune Response

Garlic, known scientifically as Allium sativum, has been used for thousands of years in both culinary and medicinal applications. It is often referred to as "nature's antibiotic" due to its potent antimicrobial, antiviral, and antifungal properties. Garlic has long been used to treat infections, boost immune function, and improve overall health.

The active compound in garlic responsible for its medicinal properties is allicin, a sulfur compound that is released when garlic is chopped or crushed. Allicin has been shown to have strong antimicrobial effects, killing or inhibiting the growth of bacteria, viruses, and fungi. Garlic has been particularly effective against respiratory infections, such as colds and flu, and is often used to fight off bacterial infections like strep throat and pneumonia.

In addition to its antibacterial properties, garlic enhances the immune response by increasing the production of white blood cells and promoting the activity of macrophages, which are cells that engulf and digest harmful pathogens. Regular consumption of garlic has also been shown to reduce the severity and duration of illnesses, improve cardiovascular health, and lower blood pressure.

Garlic can be consumed in various forms, including raw garlic, garlic powder, garlic supplements, and garlic oil. To maximize its medicinal effects, garlic is best consumed raw or lightly cooked, as heat can diminish its active compounds. For those who find the strong taste of raw garlic too potent, adding it to soups, stews, or smoothies can help integrate it into the diet.

Conclusion

The herbs and foods discussed in this chapter—echinacea, elderberry, ginger & turmeric, and garlic—offer powerful, natural support for the immune system. By incorporating these immune-boosting remedies into your daily routine, you can help to strengthen your body's defenses, prevent infections, and promote overall wellness. These herbs have been used for centuries, and their benefits are supported by modern scientific research. Whether you are looking to prevent illness, speed up recovery, or simply maintain good health, these natural remedies offer a safe, effective, and holistic way to support your body's immune system.

Chapter 4

Respiratory Health

The respiratory system is one of the body's most vital systems, responsible for delivering oxygen to the body and removing carbon dioxide. When the respiratory system becomes compromised, it can lead to discomfort, difficulty breathing, and more serious conditions like bronchitis, asthma, or pneumonia. Fortunately, nature offers many remedies to support and enhance respiratory health. In this chapter, we will explore several natural remedies that can soothe sore throats, ease congestion, and improve overall lung health. These include honey & lemon, peppermint & eucalyptus, thyme, and mullein leaf tea—all of which have been used for centuries to support respiratory well-being.

Honey & Lemon: A Soothing Remedy for Sore Throats and Coughs

Honey and lemon are two of the oldest and most trusted home remedies for respiratory issues, particularly sore throats and coughs. Both ingredients have healing properties that help to alleviate discomfort, reduce inflammation, and support the immune system.

Honey is well-known for its antimicrobial properties, thanks to its high content of natural sugars, enzymes, and antioxidants. It has a soothing effect on the throat, reducing irritation and inflammation. Honey also forms a protective coating over the throat, which helps to alleviate the constant tickling sensation that often accompanies a cough. In addition to its soothing properties, honey is rich in antioxidants, which help to fight free radicals and support the body's overall immune health.

Honey is also known for its ability to fight infections. It has been shown to be particularly effective against bacterial infections, making it an excellent choice for soothing a sore throat caused by a cold or respiratory infection. Moreover, manuka honey, a type of honey from New Zealand, is particularly potent due to its high levels of methylglyoxal, which enhances its antimicrobial and anti-inflammatory effects.

Lemon, on the other hand, is an excellent source of vitamin C, an essential nutrient that helps to boost the immune system and reduce the severity and duration of illnesses like the common cold. Lemon also has natural antiseptic properties, helping to cleanse the throat and break down mucus. The acidity of lemon juice helps to thin mucus, making it easier to expel and reducing the feeling of congestion.

Together, honey and lemon create a powerful combination for alleviating sore throats, soothing coughs, and improving respiratory health. To make a simple remedy, mix a tablespoon of honey with the juice of half a lemon in warm water. Sip this mixture slowly for maximum relief. For added benefits, you can also add a pinch of ginger powder or turmeric to enhance the anti-inflammatory effects.

Peppermint & Eucalyptus: Essential Oils for Clearing Sinuses and Easing Breathing

Peppermint and eucalyptus are two of the most widely used essential oils for promoting respiratory health. These oils have been used for centuries in traditional medicine to treat symptoms of colds, congestion, and sinus issues. Both peppermint and eucalyptus possess powerful compounds that help to clear the sinuses, open the airways, and promote easier breathing.

- Peppermint: The primary active compound in peppermint, menthol, is responsible for many of its therapeutic effects. Menthol has a cooling and soothing effect that helps to open up the airways and ease congestion. It also has antibacterial and anti-inflammatory properties, making it effective at fighting respiratory infections and reducing swelling in the airways. Additionally, peppermint is an excellent remedy for soothing a sore throat and relieving coughs due to its ability to thin mucus and facilitate expectoration.

Peppermint essential oil can be used in various ways to support respiratory health. Inhalation of steam infused with peppermint oil can help clear nasal passages and ease breathing. You can also add a few drops of peppermint essential oil to a bowl of hot water, place a towel over your head, and inhale the steam for 5–10 minutes. Another method is to dilute peppermint oil with a carrier oil, such as coconut oil or olive oil, and massage it onto the chest and throat to help relieve congestion and improve breathing.

- Eucalyptus: Eucalyptus oil is derived from the leaves of the Eucalyptus globulus tree, native to Australia. It is well-known for its powerful decongestant and expectorant properties, making it a go-to remedy for clearing the sinuses, easing breathing, and relieving symptoms of respiratory conditions like asthma, bronchitis, and the flu. The primary active compound in eucalyptus oil, eucalyptol (also known as 1,8-cineole), is responsible for its ability to relieve nasal congestion, reduce inflammation, and promote easier airflow.

Eucalyptus oil works by dilating the airways, allowing for better airflow and easier breathing. It also helps to break up mucus and encourages its expulsion, making it especially useful for people suffering from colds or respiratory infections. Like peppermint, eucalyptus essential oil can be used in steam inhalation or diffused into the air to promote respiratory health. It can also be applied topically in diluted form to the chest or back to relieve congestion and support healthy lung function.

Both peppermint and eucalyptus essential oils are valuable tools for respiratory support, especially when dealing with congestion, sinus pressure, or a cough. These oils can be used independently or together in a steam inhalation or vapor rub for optimal benefits.

Thyme: A Natural Expectorant to Relieve Congestion

Thyme (Thymus vulgaris) is a powerful herb that has been used for centuries in both culinary and medicinal practices. It is especially well-known for its ability to promote respiratory health by acting as a natural expectorant, which helps to relieve congestion and promote the expulsion of mucus from the lungs.

Thyme contains several active compounds, including thymol, which is responsible for its antimicrobial and anti-inflammatory effects. Thymol is a potent antiseptic that helps to kill bacteria and fungi in the respiratory tract, making thyme an effective herb for treating respiratory infections like bronchitis and pneumonia. Additionally, thyme has antispasmodic properties, which can help to ease coughing fits and relieve inflammation in the airways.

Thyme is a powerful herb that can help alleviate symptoms of congestion, coughing, and respiratory distress. It is particularly useful for treating bronchitis, asthma, and other conditions that involve thick mucus buildup in the lungs. One of the best ways to use thyme for respiratory health is through thyme tea.

To make thyme tea, add 1–2 teaspoons of dried thyme leaves to a cup of boiling water and steep for 5–10 minutes. Strain and sip the tea slowly for relief. If desired, you can also add honey or lemon to enhance the soothing and immune-boosting effects. Thyme can also be used in steam inhalation, as inhaling the steam from thyme tea can help to clear the sinuses and ease breathing.

For those who prefer a more concentrated form, thyme essential oil can be used in steam inhalations or diffused into the air. As with other essential oils, it's important to dilute thyme oil with a carrier oil before applying it topically, especially on sensitive skin.

Mullein Leaf Tea: A Herbal Solution for Lung and Bronchial Health

Mullein (Verbascum thapsus) is a tall, flowering plant that has been used for centuries in herbal medicine to support lung and bronchial health. Mullein is known for its soothing properties, making it an excellent remedy for treating respiratory conditions such as bronchitis, asthma, and coughs. It is particularly useful for individuals dealing with chronic respiratory conditions or those recovering from respiratory infections.

Mullein leaves contain a variety of beneficial compounds, including saponins, which act as natural expectorants to help clear mucus from the lungs. Mullein also has anti-inflammatory, antibacterial, and antiviral properties, making it effective for treating respiratory infections and promoting lung health. The leaves and flowers of the mullein plant are typically used to make mullein leaf tea, which is a gentle yet effective remedy for respiratory conditions.

Mullein tea works by soothing the respiratory tract, reducing inflammation, and helping to clear mucus from the lungs. It is particularly effective for relieving symptoms of congestion, coughing, and wheezing. To make mullein leaf tea, simply steep 1–2 teaspoons of dried mullein leaves in a cup of boiling water for 10–15 minutes. Strain the tea to remove any loose plant fibers, which can irritate the throat.

In addition to tea, mullein is also available in capsule or tincture form, which may be more convenient for those looking for a more concentrated remedy. Mullein can also be used in combination with other herbs, such as licorice root or marshmallow root, for enhanced respiratory support.

Conclusion

Respiratory health is crucial to overall well-being, and the remedies discussed in this chapter offer safe, natural alternatives to support lung and bronchial health. Honey & lemon provide soothing relief for sore throats and coughs, while peppermint & eucalyptus essential oils clear sinuses and promote easier breathing. Thyme serves as a natural expectorant, helping to expel mucus and relieve congestion, and mullein leaf tea is a gentle, effective remedy for maintaining lung health. By incorporating these natural remedies into your daily routine, you can support respiratory health, alleviate symptoms of congestion, and promote long-term lung and bronchial wellness.

Chapter 5

Digestive Health

Digestive health is at the core of overall well-being. A properly functioning digestive system ensures the body can absorb vital nutrients, eliminate waste efficiently, and maintain a strong immune system. However, digestive issues such as indigestion, bloating, constipation, and acid reflux are common complaints that can significantly impact one's quality of life. Fortunately, nature offers a range of remedies that can support and promote digestive health. In this chapter, we will explore four powerful natural solutions—ginger tea, peppermint tea, probiotics, and aloe vera—that are known for their ability to alleviate digestive discomfort, support healthy digestion, and restore balance in the gut.

Ginger Tea: A Remedy for Nausea, Indigestion, and Bloating

Ginger has been used for thousands of years in traditional medicine for its numerous health benefits, particularly for digestive health. The root of the Zingiber officinale plant contains several bioactive compounds, including gingerol and shogaol, that provide anti-inflammatory, antioxidant, and digestive-supporting properties. Ginger is especially effective for soothing nausea, alleviating indigestion, and reducing bloating.

One of the most common uses for ginger is as a remedy for nausea. Whether caused by motion sickness, pregnancy, chemotherapy, or other factors, ginger has been shown to reduce nausea and vomiting. Studies have demonstrated that ginger can be more effective than some pharmaceutical anti-nausea medications, without the side effects commonly associated with these drugs. It works by promoting the movement of food and gas through the stomach and intestines, helping to prevent nausea and vomiting.

Ginger also has a long history of use for indigestion, a condition characterized by discomfort, bloating, and fullness after eating. Ginger stimulates the production of gastric juices, which can help speed up digestion, reduce bloating, and ease the feeling of fullness. Additionally, ginger has been shown to improve gastrointestinal motility, meaning it helps move food more efficiently through the digestive tract, preventing discomfort from sluggish digestion.

Bloating is another common digestive issue that ginger can help alleviate. Bloating occurs when excess gas accumulates in the stomach and intestines, leading to feelings of discomfort and heaviness. Ginger can help reduce bloating by promoting the movement of gas and easing tension in the digestive tract.

To enjoy the digestive benefits of ginger, one of the best ways is to consume it as a ginger tea. To make ginger tea, simply peel and slice fresh ginger root and steep it in boiling water for 10–15 minutes. You can add honey or lemon to enhance the flavor and further support digestion. For those who prefer convenience, ginger powder can also be used to make tea or added to smoothies.

Peppermint Tea: Calming the Stomach and Promoting Healthy Digestion

Peppermint, or Mentha piperita, is another herb that has been widely used for centuries to support digestive health. The active compounds in peppermint, including menthol and menthone, have soothing and anti-inflammatory effects on the digestive system. Peppermint is particularly effective for calming the stomach, easing discomfort, and promoting healthy digestion.

One of the most common uses of peppermint is for relieving indigestion. Peppermint works by relaxing the muscles of the digestive tract, which helps to reduce spasms and cramping. This is particularly helpful for conditions such as irritable bowel syndrome (IBS), where abdominal pain and bloating are common symptoms. Peppermint is also effective in reducing the production of excess stomach acid, which can lead to acid reflux and heartburn. By calming the stomach and reducing irritation, peppermint tea can provide significant relief from these conditions.

Peppermint has been shown to promote gastrointestinal motility, helping food move through the digestive system more efficiently. This can help alleviate gastritis (inflammation of the stomach lining) and flatulence, both of which can cause bloating, discomfort, and pain. Peppermint is also known to help relieve nausea and reduce the sensation of fullness that accompanies indigestion.

For those suffering from gastritis or IBS, peppermint can be a helpful and gentle remedy. The cooling effect of menthol soothes the stomach lining, reducing inflammation and irritation, and calming the digestive system. Peppermint's ability to promote the flow of bile also helps in the digestion of fats, making it an excellent choice after a heavy meal.

To make peppermint tea, simply add fresh peppermint leaves or peppermint tea bags to boiling water and steep for 5–10 minutes. Drinking peppermint tea after meals can help calm the digestive system and ease discomfort. For those who prefer a more concentrated dose, peppermint essential oil can be used in a diffuser or diluted with a carrier oil and applied to the abdomen to promote digestion.

Probiotics: The Benefits of Fermented Foods for Gut Health

Probiotics are beneficial bacteria that play a crucial role in maintaining gut health. They help to restore balance to the gut microbiota, which consists of trillions of bacteria living in the intestines. A healthy gut microbiota is essential for proper digestion, nutrient absorption, and immune function. However, factors such as poor diet, stress, and the overuse of antibiotics can disrupt the balance of gut bacteria, leading to digestive issues, bloating, and even immune system problems.

Probiotics work by introducing beneficial bacteria into the gut, which helps to crowd out harmful bacteria, improve the gut lining, and support healthy digestion. These good bacteria help to break down food, absorb nutrients, and maintain the health of the gut's mucosal lining. They also play a critical role in the production of short-chain fatty acids, which are important for maintaining the integrity of the digestive tract and regulating inflammation.

Fermented foods are some of the best natural sources of probiotics. These foods are created through the process of fermentation, where beneficial bacteria are used to break down sugars and starches, producing a wide variety of beneficial microorganisms. Common fermented foods rich in probiotics include:

• Yogurt: Made from milk fermented with beneficial bacteria, yogurt is a well-known source of probiotics that supports gut health and digestion.

• Kefir: A fermented milk drink that contains a wide variety of probiotic strains, kefir is particularly effective at improving gut health and digestion.

- Sauerkraut: Fermented cabbage that is rich in beneficial bacteria, sauerkraut promotes digestive health and helps to maintain a balanced gut microbiota.

- Kimchi: A Korean fermented dish made from vegetables (typically cabbage or radishes) and seasoned with spices. Like sauerkraut, kimchi is an excellent source of probiotics.

- Kombucha: A fermented tea drink that is rich in probiotics, kombucha helps support the gut microbiota and improve digestion.

Incorporating these probiotic-rich foods into your daily diet can provide numerous digestive benefits. They help to restore balance to the gut microbiota, alleviate symptoms of indigestion and bloating, and promote regular bowel movements. Fermented foods are especially beneficial for people suffering from IBS, irritable bowel disease (IBD), and constipation, as they help regulate digestion and improve nutrient absorption.

For those who are unable to consume fermented foods, probiotic supplements are also available. These supplements provide concentrated doses of beneficial bacteria and can be an effective option for restoring gut health.

Aloe Vera: Healing the Digestive Tract and Soothing Inflammation

Aloe vera is a succulent plant known for its soothing and healing properties. It has long been used in traditional medicine to treat a variety of digestive issues, from heartburn and acid reflux to irritable bowel syndrome (IBS) and inflammatory bowel disease (IBD). The gel inside the leaves of the aloe vera plant contains a wealth of bioactive compounds, including polysaccharides, anthraquinones, and saponins, that help to heal and soothe the digestive tract.

Aloe vera has powerful anti-inflammatory properties that can help reduce irritation in the digestive tract. It is particularly useful for conditions like gastritis, ulcers, and acid reflux, where inflammation and irritation of the stomach lining can cause pain and discomfort. Aloe vera's soothing properties help to reduce this inflammation, providing relief from the burning sensation associated with heartburn and acid reflux.

In addition to its anti-inflammatory effects, aloe vera has laxative properties, making it beneficial for those suffering from constipation. The anthraquinones in aloe vera stimulate the muscles of the intestines, promoting bowel movements and easing the passage of stool. However, it's important to use aloe vera for constipation in moderation, as excessive use can lead to dehydration and electrolyte imbalances.

Aloe vera is available in several forms, including aloe vera juice, gel, and capsules. When purchasing aloe vera juice, it is important to choose a product that is free from artificial additives and preservatives. For optimal digestive health, aloe vera juice can be consumed in small amounts daily to soothe the digestive tract and support overall digestion.

Conclusion

Digestive health is crucial for overall well-being, and the remedies discussed in this chapter—ginger tea, peppermint tea, probiotics, and aloe vera—offer natural and effective ways to support the digestive system. From soothing nausea and indigestion to promoting gut health and healing inflammation, these natural remedies provide gentle and holistic solutions for common digestive issues. By incorporating these herbs and foods into your daily routine, you can promote a healthy digestive system, alleviate discomfort, and improve your overall quality of life.

Chapter 6

Skin Health and Healing

The skin is the body's largest organ and serves as the first line of defense against harmful external elements, such as bacteria, viruses, and environmental toxins. It is constantly exposed to stressors, including pollution, UV radiation, and physical trauma, which can lead to various skin issues like dryness, irritation, rashes, and infections. Thankfully, nature has provided a wide range of healing herbs and oils that can help maintain skin health and accelerate healing. In this chapter, we will explore four powerful natural remedies—aloe vera gel, calendula, lavender oil, and tea tree oil—that are known for their ability to soothe, heal, and restore the skin.

Aloe Vera Gel: A Natural Remedy for Burns, Cuts, and Skin Irritation

Aloe vera is one of the most well-known and widely used plants for skin health. For centuries, aloe vera has been prized for its soothing, hydrating, and healing properties. The gel inside the leaves of the aloe vera plant is packed with beneficial compounds, including vitamins A, C, and E, amino acids, enzymes, and polysaccharides. These compounds work together to nourish the skin, reduce inflammation, and speed up the healing process.

One of the most popular uses for aloe vera is as a remedy for burns. Whether from sun exposure, minor household burns, or friction burns, aloe vera gel is highly effective in providing relief. It works by cooling the skin, reducing the sensation of heat, and alleviating pain. The gel also promotes the regeneration of skin cells, accelerating the healing of damaged tissue. Aloe vera's anti-inflammatory properties help reduce swelling and redness, making it particularly effective for first-degree burns, mild sunburns, and scalds.

Aloe vera is also excellent for cuts and other minor wounds. The gel creates a protective barrier over the wound, keeping it hydrated and preventing infection. Its antibacterial properties help prevent microbial growth, ensuring that the wound stays clean as it heals. Aloe vera also aids in collagen production, which is essential for tissue repair and skin regeneration, allowing the skin to heal faster and more efficiently.

For skin irritation caused by conditions like eczema, psoriasis, or insect bites, aloe vera can be an incredibly soothing remedy. Its moisturizing properties help alleviate dryness and itching, while its anti-inflammatory compounds reduce redness and swelling. Aloe vera gel can be applied directly to the affected area, or it can be used in conjunction with other healing oils and creams for enhanced effects.

To use aloe vera for skin healing, simply break open a fresh aloe vera leaf and apply the gel directly to the skin. Alternatively, store-bought aloe vera gel (preferably organic and free of additives) can also be used. Aloe vera gel is gentle enough for daily use and can be applied multiple times a day as needed.

Calendula: Healing Properties for Wounds, Rashes, and Eczema

Calendula (Calendula officinalis), also known as marigold, is a beautiful, vibrant flower that has been used for centuries to promote skin health and healing. Calendula is known for its powerful anti-inflammatory, antiseptic, and antibacterial properties, making it an excellent remedy for treating wounds, rashes, eczema, and other skin conditions.

Calendula's healing powers are primarily attributed to its rich content of flavonoids and carotenoids, which possess antioxidant and anti-inflammatory effects. These compounds help to reduce swelling and redness, alleviate pain, and protect the skin from oxidative stress. Calendula has also been shown to promote collagen production, which is essential for wound healing and tissue repair.

One of the most common uses for calendula is for treating wounds. Whether it's a small cut, scrape, or more severe abrasion, calendula is excellent at speeding up the healing process. It helps prevent infection by acting as a natural antiseptic and also keeps the wound hydrated, which is essential for proper healing. Calendula also encourages the growth of new tissue, which is vital for closing up the wound and restoring the skin's integrity.

Calendula is particularly effective for skin conditions like eczema and psoriasis, which involve inflammation and irritation of the skin. It can help soothe the skin, reduce itching, and promote healing of the affected areas. Additionally, calendula's moisturizing properties make it ideal for treating dry, cracked skin, which is often a symptom of these conditions.

For rashes caused by allergic reactions, insect bites, or contact dermatitis, calendula helps reduce swelling, redness, and itching. Its gentle, soothing properties provide instant relief from irritation and discomfort.

Calendula can be used in various forms, including calendula oil, calendula-infused creams, or calendula tea. Calendula oil, in particular, can be applied directly to the skin to promote healing. Simply massage the oil onto the affected area and allow it to absorb. Calendula ointments and creams are also available and can be used as a daily treatment for irritated or inflamed skin.

Lavender Oil: Soothing for Burns, Acne, and Skin Infections

Lavender oil (Lavandula angustifolia) is one of the most versatile and widely used essential oils in natural healing. Known for its calming and soothing properties, lavender oil is an excellent remedy for a variety of skin issues, from burns and acne to infections and irritation. It has a powerful combination of antiseptic, anti-inflammatory, and antioxidant properties that make it ideal for promoting skin health and healing.

One of the most common uses of lavender oil is for treating burns. Lavender oil has been shown to promote faster healing of burns, both by reducing pain and preventing infection. The oil helps to soothe the skin, reduce redness, and stimulate cell regeneration. Lavender oil's calming effects can also help relieve the anxiety and discomfort that often accompany burns, making it an excellent choice for both emotional and physical healing.

For acne, lavender oil can be highly beneficial due to its antibacterial properties. Lavender helps fight the bacteria responsible for acne breakouts, preventing new pimples from forming. It also has an ability to balance oil production in the skin, which is particularly helpful for those with oily or combination skin. Lavender oil helps calm the skin, reducing inflammation and redness associated with acne.

Lavender oil is also useful for treating skin infections caused by bacteria, fungi, or viruses. Its antiseptic properties make it effective for treating minor skin infections such as cuts, abrasions, and insect bites. Lavender oil can prevent the growth of harmful bacteria and fungi while promoting healing and reducing the risk of scarring.

To use lavender oil for skin health, it is best to dilute it with a carrier oil (such as coconut oil, jojoba oil, or almond oil) before applying it to the skin. This helps prevent irritation and ensures safe application. You can apply the diluted oil to the affected area, or use it in a soothing lavender oil bath for general relaxation and skin rejuvenation.

Tea Tree Oil: The Antiseptic Powerhouse for Treating Acne and Fungal Infections

Tea tree oil (Melaleuca alternifolia) is a powerful essential oil known for its strong antiseptic, antifungal, and antibacterial properties. It has been used for centuries by Indigenous Australians to treat a wide range of skin issues. Tea tree oil is particularly effective for acne, fungal infections, and general skin infections.

Tea tree oil is well-known for its ability to treat acne due to its ability to kill the bacteria (specifically Propionibacterium acnes) that contribute to the development of pimples and pustules. It also helps reduce inflammation and redness associated with acne, promoting healing and preventing future breakouts. Tea tree oil works by penetrating the skin and opening clogged pores, allowing for better airflow and reducing the risk of infection.

Tea tree oil is also highly effective for treating fungal infections like athlete's foot, ringworm, and nail fungus. Its antifungal properties make it a natural and safe alternative to chemical antifungal creams, without the harsh side effects. Tea tree oil can be applied directly to the affected area, helping to reduce itching, burning, and inflammation while promoting healing of the skin.

For general skin infections, tea tree oil acts as a powerful antiseptic, preventing the growth of harmful bacteria and fungi. It can be used to treat minor cuts, abrasions, and insect bites, and is effective in reducing swelling and pain associated with these injuries.

To use tea tree oil for skin issues, dilute it with a carrier oil to prevent irritation. Apply the diluted oil to the affected area once or twice a day until the infection or acne improves. Tea tree oil is a potent remedy, so it is important to use it in moderation and always test for sensitivity before applying it to large areas of the skin.

Conclusion

The skin is a reflection of our internal health, and it requires care and attention to maintain its vitality. Natural remedies such as aloe vera gel, calendula, lavender oil, and tea tree oil offer a safe, effective, and gentle way to promote skin health and accelerate healing. Whether treating burns, cuts, acne, or skin infections, these powerful natural remedies provide relief, reduce inflammation, and support the skin's ability to regenerate. By incorporating these healing herbs and oils into your skincare routine, you can maintain healthy, radiant skin and support the body's natural healing process.

Chapter 7

Pain and Inflammation Relief

Pain and inflammation are two of the most common complaints that people experience in daily life. Whether it's chronic pain from conditions like arthritis, acute pain from an injury, or the discomfort that comes with stress and muscle tension, finding natural remedies to alleviate pain and inflammation is essential for maintaining a healthy and active lifestyle. While pharmaceuticals are often used to manage these conditions, they can come with side effects and risks. Thankfully, nature provides a variety of effective alternatives to support pain relief and reduce inflammation. In this chapter, we will explore four powerful natural remedies—turmeric & curcumin, arnica, lavender & chamomile, and willow bark—that can help manage pain, reduce inflammation, and promote healing.

Turmeric & Curcumin: The Natural Anti-Inflammatory Agents That Relieve Joint Pain

Turmeric, a bright yellow-orange root from the plant Curcuma longa, has long been used in traditional medicine, especially in Ayurveda, for its powerful anti-inflammatory and pain-relieving properties. The active compound in turmeric, curcumin, is responsible for many of its health benefits. Curcumin has been extensively studied for its ability to reduce inflammation, alleviate pain, and support overall joint and muscle health.

Inflammation is the body's natural response to injury or infection, but when it becomes chronic, it can lead to a host of health problems, including joint pain, arthritis, and even conditions like heart disease and cancer. Curcumin has been shown to work by blocking specific molecules that play a role in the inflammatory process, such as pro-inflammatory cytokines and enzymes like cyclooxygenase-2 (COX-2). By inhibiting these molecules, curcumin helps to reduce the production of inflammation-causing substances in the body.

For joint pain, particularly in conditions like osteoarthritis and rheumatoid arthritis, curcumin has been found to be highly effective in reducing pain and stiffness. Studies have shown that curcumin can help improve joint function, reduce swelling, and enhance mobility. In fact, some studies suggest that curcumin may work as effectively as non-steroidal anti-inflammatory drugs (NSAIDs), without the adverse side effects associated with these medications.

In addition to joint pain, turmeric and curcumin are also beneficial for muscle pain, as they reduce inflammation and promote tissue repair. The antioxidant properties of curcumin help to combat oxidative stress, which contributes to muscle fatigue and soreness.

One of the best ways to incorporate turmeric into your daily routine is by drinking turmeric tea or making golden milk. Golden milk is a delicious, warming beverage made with turmeric, milk (or plant-based milk), and spices like black pepper and cinnamon. Black pepper enhances the absorption of curcumin, making the remedy even more effective. Turmeric can also be taken in capsule or powder form, or added to soups, stews, and curries.

While curcumin is generally well-tolerated, its bioavailability is limited, meaning it is not easily absorbed by the body. To maximize the absorption of curcumin, it is important to consume it alongside fats (such as coconut oil) or black pepper.

Arnica: A Healing Herb for Bruises, Sprains, and Muscle Pain

Arnica (Arnica montana) is a flowering herb that has been used for centuries to treat bruises, sprains, muscle pain, and other types of physical trauma. It is particularly popular in homeopathic and herbal medicine for its ability to reduce pain, swelling, and inflammation. Arnica is most commonly applied topically in the form of creams, gels, or tinctures, but it can also be taken orally in homeopathic remedies.

Arnica contains several active compounds, including sesquiterpene lactones, which have powerful anti-inflammatory and analgesic properties. These compounds help to reduce swelling and bruising by increasing circulation to the affected area and promoting the removal of excess fluid. Arnica also works to reduce pain by blocking pain receptors and soothing the muscles.

For bruises and contusions, arnica is highly effective at speeding up the healing process.

By applying arnica topically to the bruised area, you can help to reduce discoloration, swelling, and discomfort. Arnica works by stimulating blood flow and encouraging the body to reabsorb the blood that has leaked into the tissues, which helps to heal the bruise more quickly.

Arnica is also beneficial for muscle pain and sprains. Whether you've overexerted yourself at the gym or suffered a mild sprain from an accident, arnica can provide relief. It helps to reduce the inflammation and swelling that often accompany muscle injuries and promotes faster healing by encouraging tissue repair.

To use arnica, apply an arnica gel or cream to the affected area up to three times a day. Be sure to follow the instructions on the product label, as some forms of arnica should not be applied to broken skin. Arnica should be used with caution for internal use, especially in large doses, as it can cause side effects like gastrointestinal irritation.

Lavender & Chamomile: Relaxing Oils to Relieve Tension and Stress-Related Pain

Stress is a major contributor to chronic pain, particularly tension-related pain such as headaches, neck pain, and lower back pain. When the body is under stress, muscles tense up, blood pressure rises, and inflammation increases, all of which can exacerbate pain. Lavender and chamomile are two of the most popular essential oils used for their relaxing, calming, and pain-relieving properties.

•	Lavender Oil: Lavender oil (Lavandula angustifolia) is well-known for its ability to promote relaxation and reduce stress, which in turn helps to alleviate tension and muscle pain. Lavender oil has powerful analgesic and anti-inflammatory properties that make it effective for treating both physical and emotional pain. Studies have shown that inhaling lavender essential oil can help to reduce the intensity of headaches, relieve neck and shoulder pain, and alleviate tension in the muscles.

Lavender oil also has a soothing effect on the nervous system, which makes it an excellent remedy for stress-related pain. By reducing anxiety and promoting relaxation, lavender helps to reduce the muscle tightness that often accompanies stress. Additionally, its anti-inflammatory properties help to reduce swelling and discomfort associated with conditions like arthritis and fibromyalgia.

To use lavender oil for pain relief, simply add a few drops to a diffuser to enjoy its calming aroma. You can also dilute lavender oil with a carrier oil (such as jojoba oil or coconut oil) and massage it into the affected area. For headaches, inhale the scent of lavender oil directly from the bottle or apply a small amount to the temples and forehead.

- Chamomile Oil: Chamomile (Matricaria chamomilla) is another gentle, soothing herb known for its ability to reduce pain and inflammation. Chamomile essential oil contains bisabolol, an active compound with anti-inflammatory and analgesic effects. Chamomile oil is particularly effective for treating muscle tension and headaches caused by stress.

Chamomile also has mild sedative effects, which can help to calm the nervous system and reduce the perception of pain. It is especially useful for relieving stomach pain caused by stress, such as bloating, indigestion, or cramping. Like lavender, chamomile oil can be used in a diffuser, or it can be diluted and applied to sore muscles or tension points for immediate relief.

To relieve muscle tension, mix a few drops of chamomile essential oil with a carrier oil and gently massage it into the affected area. For relaxation, a chamomile-infused bath can be incredibly soothing and effective at reducing overall tension.

Willow Bark: Nature's Aspirin for Headaches and Joint Pain Relief

Willow bark (Salix alba) has been used for centuries as a natural remedy for pain and inflammation. The bark of the willow tree contains salicin, a compound that is chemically similar to aspirin. In fact, aspirin was originally derived from salicin, making willow bark a natural, herbal alternative to synthetic pain relievers.

Willow bark is particularly effective for treating headaches, back pain, and joint pain. It works by reducing the production of prostaglandins, hormone-like substances that are involved in the inflammatory response.

By inhibiting prostaglandins, willow bark helps to reduce pain and inflammation, making it useful for conditions like arthritis and muscle pain.

For headaches, willow bark is a natural alternative to aspirin. It helps reduce the tension and inflammation that can contribute to both tension headaches and migraines. Willow bark is also effective for joint pain, especially in cases of osteoarthritis, where chronic inflammation leads to joint stiffness and discomfort.

Willow bark can be consumed in various forms, including capsules, tinctures, and tea. The recommended dosage varies depending on the form, so it is important to follow the instructions provided on the product label. Willow bark is generally well-tolerated, but it should be avoided by people who are allergic to aspirin or who are taking blood-thinning medications.

Conclusion

Pain and inflammation can significantly impact the quality of life, but natural remedies offer effective, safe, and gentle alternatives to pharmaceutical drugs. Turmeric & curcumin, arnica, lavender & chamomile, and willow bark are all powerful tools for reducing pain, alleviating inflammation, and promoting healing. By incorporating these remedies into your daily routine, you can manage chronic pain, recover from injuries, and restore balance to your body. Whether you are dealing with joint pain, muscle soreness, or stress-related discomfort, these natural solutions provide relief and support for long-term wellness.

Chapter 8

Mental Wellness and Stress Relief

In today's fast-paced world, mental wellness is more important than ever. Chronic stress, anxiety, and mental fatigue can take a toll on both the mind and the body, affecting everything from our emotional well-being to our physical health. Fortunately, nature offers a wealth of powerful herbs and remedies that can help us manage stress, promote relaxation, and improve mental clarity. In this chapter, we will explore four of the most effective natural remedies for stress relief and mental wellness: ashwagandha, lavender & chamomile, rhodiola, and lemon balm. These herbs and essential oils offer natural solutions for calming the mind, reducing anxiety, improving mood, and promoting overall mental well-being.

Ashwagandha: An Adaptogen Herb for Balancing Stress and Anxiety

Ashwagandha (Withania somnifera) is a powerful herb that has been used for thousands of years in Ayurvedic medicine to support stress relief, improve mental clarity, and enhance overall health. Known as an adaptogen, ashwagandha helps the body adapt to physical and emotional stress by regulating the stress response and bringing the body back into balance.

Adaptogens are substances that help to normalize the body's physiological functions, especially during times of stress. They work by regulating the levels of cortisol, a hormone produced by the adrenal glands in response to stress. Chronic stress often leads to elevated cortisol levels, which can cause a range of issues, including anxiety, insomnia, weight gain, and even weakened immune function. Ashwagandha helps to reduce cortisol production, leading to a more balanced response to stress.

Ashwagandha has been shown to be effective in reducing anxiety and promoting a sense of calm. Studies have demonstrated that ashwagandha can lower levels of anxiety in individuals with chronic stress by affecting the brain's neurotransmitter systems. In particular, ashwagandha helps regulate GABA (gamma-aminobutyric acid), a neurotransmitter that plays a crucial role in relaxation and reducing anxiety. By supporting the body's ability to handle stress, ashwagandha promotes emotional well-being and mental resilience.

In addition to its calming effects, ashwagandha also enhances mental clarity and cognitive function. Some studies suggest that ashwagandha may improve focus and memory, making it a great herb for individuals experiencing mental fatigue or cognitive decline.

Ashwagandha can be taken in several forms, including capsules, powder, or tinctures. To experience its full benefits, it is typically recommended to take ashwagandha consistently for several weeks. The powder can be mixed with warm milk or water, and it's often taken before bedtime to promote restful sleep and relaxation.

Lavender & Chamomile: Essential Oils for Promoting Relaxation and Sleep

Lavender (Lavandula angustifolia) and chamomile (Matricaria chamomilla) are two of the most beloved and widely used essential oils for promoting relaxation, reducing stress, and enhancing sleep quality. Both of these oils have soothing, calming properties that make them effective for mental wellness and stress relief.

- Lavender Oil: Lavender essential oil is perhaps the most popular essential oil for relaxation. Its calming effects are well-documented, and it is widely used to treat insomnia, anxiety, and stress. The active compounds in lavender oil, particularly linalool and linalyl acetate, have been shown to interact with the brain's neurotransmitters, enhancing GABA activity and promoting a sense of calm. Lavender oil can help reduce the heart rate, lower blood pressure, and relieve muscle tension, all of which are common physical symptoms of stress.

Lavender oil is especially effective for promoting sleep. It has been shown to improve sleep quality and duration by helping individuals fall asleep faster and experience deeper, more restorative sleep. The soothing scent of lavender can trigger a relaxation response in the body, which makes it an ideal oil to use before bedtime.

One of the easiest ways to use lavender oil is through aromatherapy. A few drops of lavender oil can be added to a diffuser or a cotton ball and placed near the bed. Alternatively, lavender oil can be applied topically to the temples, wrists, or the back of the neck (diluted with a carrier oil) for added relaxation. Additionally, a few drops of lavender oil in a warm bath before bedtime can provide a deeply relaxing and calming experience.

- Chamomile Oil: Chamomile essential oil is another highly effective oil for promoting relaxation and sleep. Chamomile contains bisabolol, a compound known for its soothing and anti-inflammatory properties. Like lavender, chamomile oil has a calming effect on the nervous system, making it helpful for individuals experiencing anxiety, stress, and restlessness.

Chamomile oil can help to alleviate nervous tension and promote a sense of well-being by calming the mind. It is also a natural remedy for insomnia, especially when stress and anxiety are the root causes of sleep disturbances. Chamomile oil promotes a feeling of peace and tranquility, making it an excellent choice for creating a relaxing environment before bed.

To use chamomile oil, you can diffuse it in your bedroom, apply it topically to pulse points, or add it to a warm bath. Chamomile oil blends well with other essential oils like lavender and bergamot, allowing you to create a personalized sleep-enhancing blend.

Rhodiola: A Herb That Enhances Mood and Combats Fatigue

Rhodiola (Rhodiola rosea), also known as golden root or Arctic root, is another powerful adaptogen herb that has been used for centuries to combat stress, enhance mood, and improve energy levels. Rhodiola is especially helpful for individuals experiencing mental fatigue and burnout, as it helps to reduce stress while boosting both physical and mental stamina.

One of the primary benefits of rhodiola is its ability to enhance mood and reduce symptoms of depression and anxiety. Rhodiola works by increasing the availability of key neurotransmitters, such as serotonin, dopamine, and norepinephrine, which are crucial for regulating mood and emotional well-being. By balancing these neurotransmitters, rhodiola helps to stabilize mood, improve emotional resilience, and reduce the feelings of irritability and frustration that often accompany stress.

In addition to its mood-enhancing effects, rhodiola is a natural remedy for fatigue. It helps to reduce mental and physical exhaustion by promoting the body's ability to adapt to stress and increase energy levels. Rhodiola has been shown to improve cognitive function, enhance focus, and boost memory, making it an ideal herb for individuals struggling with mental fog or cognitive decline related to stress.

Rhodiola is most commonly consumed in capsules or extract form, and it is typically taken in the morning or early afternoon to avoid disrupting sleep. For best results, rhodiola should be taken consistently over several weeks. It is generally considered safe, though it is important to consult with a healthcare provider before starting any new supplement, especially if you are on medications or have underlying health conditions.

Lemon Balm: Reduces Anxiety and Improves Cognitive Function

Lemon balm (Melissa officinalis) is a member of the mint family and is known for its calming and anti-anxiety properties. It has been used for centuries as a natural remedy for stress, anxiety, and insomnia. The active compounds in lemon balm, particularly rosmarinic acid and flavonoids, are responsible for its ability to reduce anxiety and promote relaxation.

Lemon balm is often used to help alleviate mild anxiety and restlessness. It works by enhancing the activity of GABA, a neurotransmitter that plays a key role in calming the nervous system and reducing feelings of tension. Lemon balm also helps to regulate the HPA (hypothalamic-pituitary-adrenal) axis, which is responsible for managing the body's stress response. By balancing the HPA axis, lemon balm helps the body adapt to stress and reduces feelings of anxiety and nervousness.

In addition to its anxiety-relieving effects, lemon balm is beneficial for improving cognitive function and enhancing mental clarity. Some studies have shown that lemon balm can help improve memory, focus, and alertness, making it a great herb for individuals who experience mental fatigue or cognitive decline due to stress.

Lemon balm can be consumed as a tea, tincture, or capsule. Lemon balm tea is one of the most popular ways to experience its calming effects, as it is soothing and easy to incorporate into your daily routine. A cup of lemon balm tea in the evening can help ease anxiety and promote a peaceful night's sleep.

Conclusion

Mental wellness is essential for living a balanced and healthy life. Chronic stress, anxiety, and mental fatigue can negatively impact both our emotional and physical health, but nature provides us with many powerful tools to support mental well-being. Herbs like ashwagandha, lavender & chamomile, rhodiola, and lemon balm offer natural, effective solutions for managing stress, reducing anxiety, and enhancing mood and cognitive function. By incorporating these remedies into your daily routine, you can promote relaxation, improve mental clarity, and cultivate emotional resilience, helping you to live a more peaceful and balanced life.

Chapter 9

The Role of Mindfulness in Healing

In today's world, stress, anxiety, and emotional turmoil are common challenges that can affect not only our mental well-being but also our physical health. The body and mind are intricately connected, and when the mind is overwhelmed, the body can often suffer as well. One of the most powerful tools to foster healing and restore balance is mindfulness—an ancient practice that has become increasingly recognized for its ability to promote emotional healing, reduce stress, and support overall wellness.

Mindfulness, at its core, is the practice of bringing one's attention to the present moment without judgment. It involves becoming aware of thoughts, emotions, and physical sensations as they arise and acknowledging them without reacting. This practice can be a transformative force for healing the mind, body, and spirit. In this chapter, we will explore how mindfulness practices such as meditation, deep breathing, and visualization techniques can help reduce stress, promote emotional healing, and break through mental barriers.

Practicing Meditation for Stress Relief and Emotional Healing

Meditation is one of the oldest and most well-known mindfulness practices, revered across many cultures for its calming effects and profound impact on emotional healing. Regular meditation has been scientifically shown to reduce stress, anxiety, and depression, while simultaneously enhancing emotional resilience, concentration, and self-awareness.

Meditation helps us tune into the present moment, which is particularly valuable in our fast-paced, distraction-filled world. The practice involves focusing the mind and gently guiding it back to a point of concentration when distractions arise. Whether through focusing on the breath, a mantra, or an image, meditation creates a sense of peace and stillness that allows the mind to rest and recharge. This focused attention helps to deactivate the stress response by lowering the levels of cortisol, the body's primary stress hormone. By calming the nervous system, meditation helps to reduce the physical and mental effects of stress.

There are many forms of meditation, each with its unique approach to fostering healing. Some of the most popular forms of meditation include:

•	Mindfulness Meditation: This form of meditation involves paying close attention to your breath, bodily sensations, and thoughts in a non-judgmental way. By observing the flow of thoughts and emotions without getting attached to them, practitioners learn to cultivate inner calm and emotional balance.

• Loving-Kindness Meditation (Metta): This type of meditation focuses on generating feelings of compassion and goodwill toward oneself and others. Practitioners begin by directing loving-kindness toward themselves, then gradually extending it to loved ones, acquaintances, and even those with whom they may have difficulty. This practice has been shown to enhance emotional healing by promoting feelings of warmth, acceptance, and connection.

• Guided Meditation: This involves following a pre-recorded or live guide who leads you through a meditation session. Guided meditations can be focused on various aspects of healing, such as stress relief, emotional healing, or overcoming specific mental barriers. The guide's soothing voice helps to deepen relaxation and lead the practitioner toward a sense of peace.

For emotional healing, meditation helps by creating space for us to process emotions without judgment or reactivity. It allows us to sit with our feelings of sadness, grief, or anxiety without the need to escape them. In doing so, we can release pent-up emotions, gain clarity, and cultivate a more peaceful, balanced state of mind.

The healing power of meditation is cumulative. The more regularly one meditates, the more likely the benefits will be felt over time. Even just 10–20 minutes a day can significantly improve emotional well-being.

Deep Breathing Exercises to Activate the Parasympathetic Nervous System

Breathing is a vital physiological process that we often take for granted. However, breath is also a powerful tool for managing stress and promoting emotional healing. Deep breathing exercises, particularly those designed to activate the parasympathetic nervous system, can help calm the mind, reduce stress, and support physical healing by encouraging the body to shift from the "fight or flight" response into a more relaxed state.

The autonomic nervous system (ANS) regulates many involuntary bodily functions, including heart rate, digestion, and respiratory rate. The ANS is divided into two branches:

1. Sympathetic Nervous System (SNS): This system is responsible for the body's "fight or flight" response, which occurs during times of stress or danger. It increases heart rate, dilates the pupils, and prepares the body for quick action. While this response is essential for survival, prolonged

activation due to chronic stress can have detrimental effects on health.

2. Parasympathetic Nervous System (PNS): In contrast, the PNS is responsible for the "rest and digest" state, which calms the body and promotes healing. The PNS lowers the heart rate, reduces blood pressure, and encourages a sense of relaxation and well-being.

Deep breathing exercises, specifically those that emphasize slow, diaphragmatic breathing, can activate the PNS and promote a relaxation response. By consciously focusing on deep, slow breaths, we can shift our bodies out of the state of tension and anxiety that is often triggered by stress. Some popular deep breathing exercises include:

• Diaphragmatic Breathing (Belly Breathing): This involves breathing deeply into the diaphragm rather than shallowly into the chest. Place one hand on the chest and the other on the abdomen. As you inhale through the nose, allow the belly to rise, expanding with air. Exhale slowly through the mouth, letting the belly fall. This technique encourages relaxation by fully engaging the diaphragm and helping to slow the heart rate.

- 4-7-8 Breathing: This technique involves inhaling for 4 seconds, holding the breath for 7 seconds, and exhaling for 8 seconds. The extended exhalation activates the parasympathetic nervous system, promoting deep relaxation. This is particularly useful for managing stress or anxiety in the moment.

- Box Breathing: Also known as square breathing, this technique involves inhaling for a count of 4 seconds, holding for 4 seconds, exhaling for 4 seconds, and holding the breath for another 4 seconds. Box breathing is excellent for cultivating calm and can be done anytime you need to ground yourself during stressful situations.

By practicing deep breathing regularly, we can improve our ability to manage stress and shift our body into a state of healing. Deep breathing helps lower cortisol levels, reduce heart rate, and relax muscle tension, creating a sense of balance and emotional clarity.

Visualization Techniques for Healing and Overcoming Mental Barriers

Visualization, also known as guided imagery, is a powerful technique that involves imagining a specific scene, object, or situation in the mind to bring about a desired emotional or physical state. This technique is widely used in meditation and mindfulness practices to promote relaxation, reduce stress, and support healing. By using the mind to visualize positive outcomes, individuals can shift their emotional state, foster healing, and overcome mental barriers that may be hindering their progress.

Visualization works on the principle that the mind and body are closely connected. What we imagine in our minds can have a profound effect on our physical state. When we visualize positive scenarios, such as healing, success, or peace, the brain reacts as if those scenarios are real, triggering physical and emotional responses that help bring about those desired results.

There are several types of visualization techniques that can be particularly helpful in the context of healing:

- Healing Visualization: In this form of visualization, you imagine the body's immune system or healing processes at work, repairing injury or illness. For example, you might visualize a healing light moving through the body, repairing damaged cells and restoring health. This can be particularly useful for those dealing with chronic pain, illness, or emotional trauma. By mentally visualizing healing, you can increase feelings of hope, positivity, and relaxation.

• Positive Outcome Visualization: This technique focuses on visualizing a positive outcome in a specific situation. For example, if you are preparing for a stressful event, such as a presentation or an important meeting, you might visualize yourself succeeding with confidence, composure, and ease. This can help reduce anxiety, increase self-esteem, and improve your performance.

• Overcoming Mental Barriers: Many people face mental barriers that limit their ability to achieve their goals or heal. These barriers may include self-doubt, fear, or limiting beliefs. Through visualization, you can mentally overcome these barriers by seeing yourself moving past them. Imagine a scenario where you are confidently breaking through obstacles and achieving your goals. By reinforcing this positive imagery, you can begin to dismantle mental barriers and increase your belief in your ability to succeed.

Visualization techniques are incredibly versatile and can be tailored to specific needs. To practice visualization, find a quiet space where you can relax without distractions. Close your eyes and take a few deep breaths. Begin by visualizing a peaceful, positive scene—whether it's an image of health, success, or tranquility. Focus on the colors, sounds, and sensations of the scene, allowing it to envelop you completely. This practice can be done daily, particularly in moments of stress, and can serve as a powerful tool for emotional healing and self-empowerment.

Conclusion

Mindfulness practices such as meditation, deep breathing, and visualization are incredibly powerful tools for healing the mind, body, and spirit. These techniques not only reduce stress and anxiety but also promote emotional healing, mental clarity, and physical well-being. By incorporating mindfulness into our daily routines, we can cultivate a deeper sense of peace, resilience, and balance in our lives. Whether you're looking to reduce stress, overcome mental barriers, or simply promote a sense of calm and well-being, mindfulness offers a proven path toward healing and self-discovery. With consistent practice, these techniques can help you achieve emotional freedom, enhance your mental health, and support your body's natural ability to heal.

Chapter 10

Restorative Practices for the Body and Spirit

In a world where the demands of daily life often lead to physical exhaustion, mental burnout, and emotional fatigue, restorative practices can provide the necessary space to rejuvenate the body, mind, and spirit. These practices are not merely about relaxation but are deeply connected to holistic healing, helping us restore balance, increase vitality, and promote well-being. Through practices like yoga and stretching, the use of essential oils for relaxation and grounding, and spending time in nature through outdoor activities, we can tap into the body's natural ability to heal, unwind, and reconnect with ourselves.

In this chapter, we will explore how these restorative practices can support overall health and wellness, offering profound benefits for both the physical body and the spiritual self.

The Power of Yoga and Stretching for Physical and Mental Rejuvenation

Yoga is one of the most powerful practices for restoring balance to the body and mind. Rooted in ancient traditions, yoga is a holistic discipline that combines physical postures (asanas), controlled breathing techniques (pranayama), meditation, and a philosophical approach to life. The practice of yoga works on multiple levels, enhancing physical flexibility, strength, and stamina while also fostering mental clarity, emotional resilience, and spiritual growth.

• Physical Rejuvenation: On a physical level, yoga and stretching have numerous benefits. By incorporating a series of stretches and poses, yoga improves flexibility, joint mobility, and muscle strength. As the body is gently stretched and held in various positions, tension is released from the muscles, ligaments, and tendons. This release helps to improve posture, alleviate muscle stiffness, and increase circulation, allowing for better oxygen and nutrient delivery to the tissues. Regular practice can reduce the risk of injuries, improve body alignment, and relieve chronic pain caused by conditions such as arthritis or lower back pain.

Stretching through yoga also promotes detoxification. As muscles are stretched, the body encourages the flow of lymphatic fluid, which helps flush out toxins and waste products from the tissues. The deep breathing associated with yoga increases oxygenation of the cells, allowing them to work more efficiently and promoting a sense of vitality.

- Mental Rejuvenation: Yoga is just as effective for calming the mind and restoring mental clarity. The practice of mindfulness, which is an integral part of yoga, encourages present-moment awareness and helps practitioners become more attuned to their thoughts, emotions, and bodily sensations. This mental clarity can help alleviate anxiety, stress, and mental fatigue, creating a profound sense of relaxation and peace.

One of the key aspects of yoga that helps promote mental rejuvenation is breathing exercises (pranayama). The deliberate control of breath helps to activate the parasympathetic nervous system, which is responsible for the body's relaxation response. By engaging in deep, slow breathing, yoga practitioners can calm their nervous system, reduce cortisol levels (the stress hormone), and foster a sense of balance and tranquility. Some common breathing techniques, such as Ujjayi breath or Alternate Nostril Breathing, are particularly beneficial for promoting relaxation and mental clarity.

- Spiritual Rejuvenation: Yoga is not only a physical or mental practice but also a spiritual one. The practice encourages self-reflection, mindfulness, and connection to the inner self. By incorporating meditation and breath awareness, yoga helps individuals develop a deeper sense of spiritual peace, contentment, and connection to the world around them.

Yoga as a restorative practice can be as gentle as needed. Restorative yoga, which involves supported poses held for longer durations with the use of props (like blankets and blocks), is particularly beneficial for those looking to deeply relax and unwind. This practice encourages the body to surrender to gravity, allowing for profound relaxation and restoration. Gentle yoga poses, combined with breath awareness, activate the body's parasympathetic nervous system, reducing stress and promoting healing.

Whether you practice intense vinyasa flow or gentle restorative poses, yoga offers an incredible pathway for healing on all levels: physically, mentally, and spiritually.

Essential Oils for Relaxation and Spiritual Grounding

Essential oils have been used for centuries across cultures for their healing and therapeutic properties. These concentrated plant extracts, derived from flowers, herbs, seeds, and roots, are rich in aromatic compounds that can have profound effects on both the body and the spirit. Essential oils can help to reduce stress, alleviate physical discomfort, enhance mental clarity, and promote spiritual grounding.

- Lavender: Lavender essential oil is one of the most widely known and used oils for relaxation. Its calming properties make it an ideal oil for relieving stress and anxiety, promoting deep relaxation, and improving sleep quality. Lavender works by interacting with the brain's limbic system, which controls emotions and stress responses. Simply diffusing lavender oil or applying it to pulse points can help promote a sense of calm and tranquility. For spiritual grounding, lavender is also believed to help open the heart chakra, encouraging emotional balance and peacefulness.

- Frankincense: Frankincense essential oil is a powerful oil for spiritual grounding and mindfulness. It has a rich, earthy aroma that has been used in religious rituals and meditation practices for centuries. Frankincense oil helps to deepen meditation, promote emotional healing, and create a sense of peace and connection. It has the ability to calm the mind, reduce stress, and clear negative energy. Frankincense is also known for its ability to support the immune system and reduce inflammation in the body. It can be used in a diffuser, applied topically (diluted with a carrier oil), or added to a relaxing bath.

- Bergamot: Bergamot oil, derived from the peel of the citrus fruit, is an uplifting and grounding oil that helps reduce anxiety and improve mood. Its refreshing and invigorating scent can energize the mind, relieve tension, and uplift the spirit. Bergamot oil is particularly useful for balancing emotions and is often used to reduce feelings of nervousness or low energy. It is also helpful for improving focus and clarity, which can aid in mindfulness practices or meditation.

- Sandalwood: Sandalwood is a calming and centering oil that is often used in spiritual practices to promote grounding and connection to the earth. Its grounding properties make it ideal for meditation, mindfulness, and deep relaxation. Sandalwood essential oil is known for its ability to calm the nervous system, reduce stress, and promote feelings of peace. It can be diffused, applied to the chakras, or used in a bath for emotional balance and relaxation.

Essential oils can be used in a variety of ways, depending on the desired effect. Diffusing them in the air is one of the most common methods, allowing the aroma to permeate the room and create a peaceful atmosphere. You can also dilute essential oils with a carrier oil (such as coconut or jojoba oil) and apply them directly to the skin for a calming effect or use them in a warm bath for total relaxation.

Using essential oils in combination with other restorative practices like yoga or meditation can deepen the experience, providing a multi-sensory approach to healing and relaxation.

The Importance of Nature and Outdoor Activities in Holistic Health

Spending time in nature is an incredibly powerful practice for rejuvenating the body, mind, and spirit. In our modern, technology-driven world, we often become disconnected from the natural world, spending much of our time indoors or glued to screens. However, research has shown that time spent outdoors can have significant benefits for our physical and mental health.

•	Physical Benefits: Being outdoors encourages physical movement, whether it's walking, hiking, or simply spending time in a natural environment. Outdoor activities like walking in the park, hiking through forests, or swimming in lakes are excellent ways to engage in gentle exercise while benefiting from the fresh air and natural surroundings.

These activities help improve cardiovascular health, enhance muscle tone, and boost energy levels. Exposure to natural light also regulates our circadian rhythms, promoting better sleep and higher energy levels throughout the day.

- Mental and Emotional Benefits: Nature has a profound impact on mental health. Studies have shown that spending time in natural environments can reduce symptoms of stress, anxiety, and depression. Being surrounded by greenery and natural landscapes helps to calm the nervous system, promote relaxation, and create a sense of peace. This is particularly important for emotional healing, as nature allows individuals to disconnect from daily stressors and reconnect with themselves.

Time in nature also promotes mindfulness. When walking through a forest, sitting by the ocean, or hiking in the mountains, we are naturally attuned to the sights, sounds, and sensations around us. The practice of being present in nature allows us to cultivate mindfulness without needing to focus on anything but the natural world. This presence helps to ground us, reduce stress, and restore our mental clarity.

- Spiritual Benefits: Nature is deeply connected to spirituality. For many, spending time outdoors is a form of spiritual practice, whether it's connecting with the earth, engaging in meditative walks, or simply reflecting in solitude. Nature provides a profound sense of connection to something greater than ourselves, allowing us to experience a deeper sense of belonging and peace. Being in nature can help us feel grounded, clear-minded, and spiritually nourished.

Whether you're practicing yoga in the park, hiking in the mountains, or simply taking a walk through your local neighborhood, spending time outdoors is a powerful tool for holistic health. Nature provides the perfect setting for relaxation, reflection, and rejuvenation.

Conclusion

Restorative practices are essential for maintaining balance, vitality, and well-being. Yoga and stretching help rejuvenate the body and calm the mind, while essential oils promote relaxation and spiritual grounding. Spending time in nature offers profound benefits for physical, mental, and emotional health, encouraging healing on all levels. By incorporating these practices into our daily lives, we can create space for healing, reduce stress, and restore harmony between our body, mind, and spirit. Through these restorative practices, we can nurture ourselves and unlock the body's natural ability to heal, rejuvenate, and thrive.

Chapter 11

Creating a Healing Space
Building a Natural Healing Practice at Home

Creating a nurturing, healing environment in the comfort of your own home can significantly enhance both physical and emotional well-being. By incorporating natural elements and remedies into your living space, you can cultivate an atmosphere conducive to rest, relaxation, and rejuvenation. In this section, we'll explore how to design a healing space, the benefits of natural elements such as plants, crystals, and sound therapy, and how to incorporate healing herbs and remedies into your daily routine. We will also delve into providing safe and effective natural remedies for families, from children to the elderly, and how to build a natural medicine cabinet filled with essential herbs and oils. Additionally, we will discuss ways to involve the whole family in maintaining wellness through natural practices.

How to Design a Nurturing Environment for Rest and Recovery

The environment in which we spend our time has a profound effect on our physical and emotional health. A healing space is one that fosters calm, tranquility, and relaxation, offering a respite from the chaos and stress of daily life. Whether you are designing a dedicated healing room, a cozy corner for meditation, or simply transforming your entire home into a sanctuary, there are key elements you can incorporate to create an environment that supports rest and recovery.

1. Choose Calming Colors: Colors play an important role in influencing mood and energy levels. To create a soothing atmosphere, opt for soft, muted tones such as pastel blues, greens, lavender, and beige.

These colors have been shown to promote relaxation, reduce anxiety, and create a sense of calm. If you prefer a more vibrant environment, use colors that evoke feelings of warmth and joy, such as soft yellows or light oranges, while avoiding overly stimulating colors like bright reds or neon shades.

2. Declutter and Organize: A cluttered space can contribute to stress, distraction, and feelings of chaos. To create a nurturing environment, take the time to declutter your living space and organize your belongings. Keep only what serves a purpose or brings joy into your space, and create designated areas for relaxation and recovery. A minimalist approach, where everything has its place, can help bring a sense of calm to the environment.

3. Lighting and Ambiance: The right lighting can make a significant difference in

the mood of your space. Natural light is ideal for creating a healing environment. If possible, arrange your furniture to maximize exposure to natural sunlight. In spaces where natural light is limited, consider incorporating soft, ambient lighting, such as floor lamps, candles, or Himalayan salt lamps. These types of lighting are gentle on the eyes and help create a calm and restful atmosphere. Avoid harsh, overhead fluorescent lights, which can be stressful and uninviting.

4. Comfortable Furniture and Textiles: Choose furniture that promotes comfort and relaxation. Soft, cushioned chairs, couches, and pillows are perfect for creating a cozy, nurturing environment. Throw blankets, soft rugs, and cushions add warmth and texture to the room, making it a space where you can unwind completely. If you have a meditation or yoga space, incorporate a

comfortable mat or cushion to help support your practice.

5. Air Quality: Clean, fresh air is essential for creating a healing space. Poor air quality can lead to fatigue, headaches, and respiratory discomfort. To improve air quality in your home, open windows when possible to allow fresh air to circulate. Consider using an air purifier to remove dust, allergens, and toxins. Essential oils like eucalyptus, peppermint, and lemon can help purify the air while providing calming or invigorating effects. Houseplants can also improve air quality by absorbing toxins and releasing oxygen.

6. Create a Sensory Experience: Engage all of the senses to foster relaxation and healing. Use essential oils, soothing music, and textured fabrics to create an immersive environment. Place scented candles, diffusers, or incense in the room to introduce

calming fragrances like lavender, chamomile, and sandalwood. Soft instrumental music, nature sounds, or binaural beats can further enhance the atmosphere by promoting deep relaxation and focus.

7. Personalized Healing Touches: Finally, personalize your space with meaningful items that promote a sense of comfort and connection. This could include favorite books, meaningful artwork, family photographs, or spiritual items like crystals, statues, or sacred objects. Surrounding yourself with things that bring joy and calmness will create a space that feels safe and nurturing.

The Benefits of Natural Elements

1. Plants: Bringing nature indoors is one of the simplest yet most effective ways to enhance the healing power of a space. Plants purify the air, improve humidity levels, and contribute to a sense of peace and connection to the natural world. Some

plants, such as snake plants, peace lilies, and spider plants, are known for their ability to filter toxins from the air. Additionally, caring for plants can have therapeutic benefits, providing a sense of purpose and connection to life.

Plants like lavender and aloe vera can also offer medicinal benefits. Lavender's calming scent is ideal for reducing stress, while aloe vera's gel is known for its healing properties when applied to the skin. Incorporating these plants into your healing space can create an environment that nurtures both body and soul.

2. Crystals: Crystals have long been used for their healing properties, and they can help amplify the energy of your healing space. Each type of crystal is believed to have unique properties that can promote physical, emotional, or spiritual healing. For example, amethyst is often used to promote

calm and relaxation, rose quartz enhances emotional healing and self-love, and clear quartz is used to amplify energy and bring clarity. Placing crystals around your home can help harmonize the energy in the space and support your wellness practices.

3. Sound Therapy: Sound therapy, also known as sound healing, uses sound frequencies to promote healing and balance. One of the most accessible forms of sound therapy is the use of calming music or nature sounds, which can help reduce stress and anxiety. Binaural beats, which use different frequencies in each ear to create a sense of relaxation and focus, are also a powerful tool for mindfulness and meditation. You can also incorporate singing bowls, chimes, or even drumming into your space to enhance the therapeutic benefits of sound.

Incorporating Healing Herbs and Remedies into Your Daily Routine

Incorporating healing herbs and natural remedies into your daily routine is one of the most effective ways to support both your physical and emotional well-being. From morning teas to evening baths, there are numerous ways to use natural remedies to promote healing throughout your day. Here are some ideas:

1. Herbal Teas: Drinking herbal teas is one of the simplest ways to experience the benefits of healing herbs. Teas made from herbs like chamomile, ginger, peppermint, and lemongrass can help with digestion, relaxation, and immune support. Start your day with a calming cup of lavender tea to set a peaceful tone, or sip ginger tea in the afternoon for an energy boost and digestive support. You can also experiment with custom blends by combining different herbs based on your needs.

2. Herbal Infusions and Tinctures: Herbal infusions and tinctures are more concentrated than teas and can provide a powerful remedy for various health issues. For example, echinacea tincture can support immune health, while st. john's wort can be used to manage symptoms of mild depression and anxiety. Adding these concentrated forms of herbs into your daily wellness routine can provide ongoing support for your health.

3. Topical Herbal Remedies: Many herbs can also be applied topically to soothe the skin and promote healing. Aloe vera, calendula, and arnica are particularly useful for treating skin irritations, bruises, and inflammation. Create soothing lotions or balms by infusing herbs like lavender or tea tree oil in carrier oils such as coconut or olive oil. These remedies can be applied daily for their calming and healing effects.

4. Herbal Baths: Adding herbs to your bath can provide both physical and emotional healing. Epsom salts, lavender, chamomile, and rosemary are great for promoting relaxation and soothing sore muscles. To create a healing bath, simply add a handful of dried herbs or an essential oil blend to the warm water. The steam from the herbs will allow their medicinal properties to be inhaled, while the water soothes and relaxes the body.

Chapter 12: Natural Remedies for Families

Safe and Effective Herbal Remedies for Children and Elderly Care

When it comes to caring for the health and well-being of children and elderly family members, it is important to choose remedies that are gentle, safe, and effective. Many herbs that are beneficial for adults can also be used for children and the elderly, but proper dosage and precautions are crucial.

1. For Children: Children have more sensitive bodies and developing systems, so the use of herbal remedies must be approached with care. Some safe and effective herbs for children include:

o Chamomile: Chamomile tea or a chamomile-infused bath is a gentle remedy for calming children and relieving mild discomfort such as teething pain, stomachaches, or mild colic. Chamomile is a mild sedative, helping children relax before bedtime.

o Ginger: Ginger is great for relieving nausea and digestive upset. You can offer children a small amount of ginger tea, or use ginger in tincture or syrup form to soothe tummy troubles.

o Lavender: Lavender is a wonderful herb for calming anxiety, improving sleep, and reducing restlessness. Lavender essential oil can be used in a diffuser, or a few drops can be applied to the pillow to encourage peaceful sleep.

2. For the Elderly: The elderly often experience unique health challenges such as joint pain, reduced immune function, and sleep difficulties. Some herbs that are safe and effective for elderly care include:

o Turmeric: Turmeric, especially in its bioavailable curcumin form, can help reduce inflammation and support joint health. It is particularly beneficial for seniors with arthritis or other inflammatory conditions.

o Ginseng: Ginseng is a great herb for boosting energy, improving cognitive function, and supporting overall vitality. It can help combat fatigue and improve mood in the elderly.

o Valerian Root: Valerian is useful for promoting sleep and reducing anxiety. It is a safe, non-habit-forming herb that can be beneficial for seniors who struggle with insomnia or restless nights.

Building a Natural Medicine Cabinet

Having a well-stocked natural medicine cabinet is a great way to ensure that you and your family have access to safe and effective remedies for everyday ailments. Essential herbs and oils to include in your natural medicine cabinet for family use are:

•	Echinacea: For boosting the immune system and fighting off colds.

•	Arnica: For treating bruises, sprains, and muscle aches.

•	Peppermint: For digestive support, headaches, and muscle relaxation.

•	Lavender: For stress relief, sleep support, and skin healing.

•	Tea Tree Oil: For antimicrobial use, skin conditions, and cuts.

- Chamomile: For digestive issues, relaxation, and soothing skin.

How to Involve Your Family in Maintaining Wellness Through Natural Practices

Building a natural healing practice at home can be a wonderful opportunity to involve the whole family in maintaining wellness. Encourage children to participate in creating healthy meals using fresh herbs and spices, teach them about the benefits of herbal teas, or make a family ritual of practicing yoga or stretching together. By integrating natural practices into your daily routine, you not only nurture your family's physical health but also promote emotional and spiritual well-being. Incorporating mindfulness practices such as meditation or nature walks can further create a sense of connection and peace in your home.

Conclusion

Creating a nurturing and healing environment at home, incorporating herbal remedies, and involving your family in maintaining wellness are powerful steps toward holistic health. Whether it's designing a peaceful space with natural elements, building a natural medicine cabinet, or involving your loved ones in healing practices, these actions support long-term wellness for both the body and the spirit. By cultivating a healing space and embracing natural remedies, you can foster a harmonious, balanced life for yourself and your family, promoting health, happiness, and vitality in every aspect of life.

Chapter 12

Prevention through Natural Healing

Maintaining Long-Term Health and Wellness

The journey to maintaining long-term health and wellness goes beyond addressing ailments when they arise—it's about creating and sustaining a proactive, preventive approach to overall well-being. Through a combination of routine practices, self-care, mindfulness, and regular use of natural healing methods, you can cultivate a life that minimizes the risk of illness and maximizes vitality. In this section, we will explore how to build a routine that helps prevent common ailments and chronic diseases, the importance of regular herbal detoxes and cleanses, maintaining emotional well-being, and how to embrace the future of natural healing through modern advancements and holistic living.

Building a Routine to Prevent Common Ailments and Chronic Diseases

Prevention is the cornerstone of long-term health and wellness. Instead of waiting for illness to strike, it is much more beneficial to focus on building a lifestyle that supports your body's natural defenses. A regular routine that incorporates preventive measures can help ward off common ailments such as colds, digestive issues, fatigue, and even chronic diseases like heart disease, diabetes, and hypertension.

1. Daily Habits for Health:

o Hydration: One of the simplest and most effective preventive practices is ensuring that your body stays properly hydrated. Water is essential for all cellular functions and helps detoxify the body by flushing out waste products. Aim for at least 8 glasses of water a day, more if you are active or live in a hot climate.

o   Movement: Regular physical activity is vital for maintaining long-term health. Exercise strengthens the heart, supports the immune system, and helps prevent conditions like obesity, hypertension, and type 2 diabetes. Incorporating activities such as yoga, walking, swimming, or strength training into your daily routine helps maintain physical health and improves mood by releasing endorphins.

o   Sleep: Consistently getting enough restorative sleep is crucial for the prevention of illness. Poor sleep can weaken the immune system, impair cognitive function, and increase the risk of chronic diseases. Aim for 7-9 hours of quality sleep each night to allow the body time to repair and rejuvenate.

o   Stress Management: Chronic stress is one of the primary contributors to many health issues, including heart disease, high blood pressure, and digestive problems.

Practices such as mindfulness, meditation, deep breathing, and journaling can help you manage stress and improve mental well-being, which in turn supports physical health.

2. Nutrition and Lifestyle Choices: A well-balanced diet rich in nutrients is crucial for preventing illness. Focus on a diet that includes:

o Whole foods: Fruits, vegetables, whole grains, and legumes should form the foundation of your diet. These foods are rich in fiber, vitamins, and minerals that support the immune system and protect against chronic diseases.

o Healthy fats: Incorporate omega-3 fatty acids found in foods like salmon, flaxseeds, and walnuts to reduce inflammation and support brain health. Healthy fats also play a key role in maintaining hormonal balance.

o   Protein: Protein is essential for muscle repair and immune function. Sources of lean protein include chicken, tofu, beans, and lentils.

o   Spices and herbs: Many herbs and spices have anti-inflammatory and antioxidant properties that support overall health. Turmeric, ginger, garlic, cayenne pepper, and rosemary are just a few examples of powerful herbs that support immunity, reduce inflammation, and promote detoxification.

3.   Prevention of Common Ailments:

o   Cold and Flu: Regular hand washing, adequate hydration, and a diet rich in immune-boosting vitamins like Vitamin C (from citrus fruits, strawberries, and bell peppers) and Vitamin D (from sunlight or supplements) can prevent the onset of colds and flu. Echinacea and elderberry are two powerful herbs that can prevent viral infections when taken at the first signs of illness.

o	Digestive Health: A healthy digestive system is essential for overall health. Eating a fiber-rich diet, drinking plenty of water, and incorporating probiotics (found in fermented foods like yogurt, kefir, and sauerkraut) can promote healthy digestion. Herbal teas made from peppermint, ginger, or chamomile can soothe the stomach and alleviate digestive discomfort.

o	Mental Health: Regular mindfulness meditation, deep breathing exercises, and engaging in hobbies or physical activities can help manage stress and improve emotional well-being. Ashwagandha and rhodiola are two adaptogenic herbs that support the body's ability to cope with stress, reducing the risk of anxiety and depression.

The Importance of Regular Herbal Detoxes and Cleanses

Herbal detoxes and cleanses are a powerful tool for maintaining long-term health and well-being. Over time, our bodies accumulate toxins from the environment, food, and stress. These toxins can contribute to fatigue, poor digestion, and weakened immunity, making it harder for the body to heal. By regularly engaging in herbal detoxes and cleanses, you can support the body's natural detoxification processes, promote energy, and improve overall wellness.

1. Understanding Detoxification: The body has several natural detoxification systems, including the liver, kidneys, skin, and lymphatic system. These organs work to filter and eliminate toxins from the body. However, due to lifestyle factors such as poor diet, lack of exercise, environmental pollutants, and chronic stress, the body's detoxification systems can become

overburdened. Regular detox practices can help support and strengthen these systems, allowing the body to function at its optimal level.

2.	Herbal Detox Programs:

o	Dandelion Root: Known for its liver-supporting properties, dandelion root helps stimulate bile production, which aids in the breakdown and elimination of toxins. It also supports the kidneys by promoting urination and flushing out excess fluids and waste.

o	Milk Thistle: This powerful herb is widely recognized for its ability to detoxify and regenerate the liver. Silymarin, the active compound in milk thistle, helps protect liver cells from damage and promotes healthy liver function.

o	Cilantro: Cilantro is known for its ability to help the body detox heavy metals such as mercury, aluminum, and lead. It binds to these metals and helps eliminate them through the digestive tract.

o   Lemon Water: Drinking warm water with freshly squeezed lemon in the morning helps stimulate digestion, hydrate the body, and promote the detoxification process. Lemon juice contains high levels of Vitamin C, which supports the liver's detoxifying functions.

3.   Cleansing Herbs for Digestive Health:

o   Psyllium Husk: Psyllium husk is a fiber-rich herb that helps cleanse the colon and support digestive health. It works by absorbing water and forming a gel-like substance that helps to eliminate waste from the intestines, promoting regular bowel movements.

o   Ginger and Turmeric: Both of these herbs have anti-inflammatory properties that support digestive health and reduce bloating, gas, and indigestion. They also promote the movement of bile, which aids in fat digestion.

4. The Benefits of Fasting: While herbal detoxes can be done daily or weekly, fasting is another powerful practice that supports the body's natural detoxification processes. Fasting allows the body time to rest, repair, and eliminate toxins. Intermittent fasting, which involves cycling between periods of eating and fasting, can have profound health benefits, including improving metabolism, supporting the liver, and promoting cell repair.

Maintaining Emotional Well-Being through Balanced Nutrition and Self-Care

Emotional health is just as important as physical health when it comes to long-term wellness. Chronic stress, anxiety, and emotional imbalances can take a toll on the body, contributing to digestive issues, hormonal imbalances, and weakened immunity. One of the best ways to maintain emotional well-being is by focusing on balanced nutrition, self-care, and cultivating emotional resilience.

1.   Balanced Nutrition for Emotional Health:

o   Omega-3 Fatty Acids: These essential fats, found in fatty fish, flaxseeds, and walnuts, support brain function and help manage mood. Low levels of omega-3 fatty acids have been linked to mood disorders such as depression and anxiety.

o   Magnesium: Magnesium is a mineral that plays a crucial role in reducing stress and supporting the nervous system. It helps regulate the production of stress hormones and promotes relaxation. Foods rich in magnesium include leafy greens, almonds, and dark chocolate.

o   B Vitamins: B vitamins, particularly B6, B12, and folate, are essential for maintaining a healthy nervous system and balanced mood. These vitamins are found in whole grains, legumes, leafy greens, and eggs.

o   Probiotics: The gut-brain connection is a key factor in emotional health. A healthy gut microbiome supports the production of neurotransmitters like serotonin, which regulates mood and emotional well-being. Eating foods rich in probiotics, such as yogurt, kimchi, and kombucha, can improve gut health and help manage stress.

2.   Self-Care Practices for Emotional Healing:

o   Mindfulness and Meditation: Regular mindfulness practice helps you manage stress, reduce negative thoughts, and increase emotional awareness. Meditation also promotes relaxation by lowering cortisol levels and activating the parasympathetic nervous system.

o	Journaling: Journaling is a therapeutic tool that allows you to express emotions, reflect on your experiences, and process difficult feelings. Regular journaling can help release pent-up emotions, gain clarity, and foster a sense of calm.

o	Creative Expression: Engaging in creative activities such as art, music, or writing can provide an emotional outlet and help alleviate stress. Creative practices can help you tap into your emotions, reduce anxiety, and boost overall well-being.

Chapter 13

Embracing the Future of Natural Healing

Modern Advancements in Herbal Medicine and Integrative Health

The future of natural healing is exciting, with ongoing advancements in herbal medicine, integrative health practices, and holistic approaches to wellness. Modern science continues to validate the effectiveness of traditional herbal remedies, while also providing new insights into how plants and natural substances interact with the body's systems.

1. Scientific Research on Herbs: As interest in herbal medicine grows, more studies are being conducted to explore the effectiveness of various herbs in treating a wide range of health conditions. Researchers are uncovering new active compounds and understanding how these compounds interact

with the body's cells and organs. For example, research on curcumin, the active compound in turmeric, has shown promising results in treating inflammation, pain, and even cancer.

2. Integrative Health Approaches: Integrative medicine combines conventional medical treatments with alternative therapies such as acupuncture, herbal remedies, and mind-body practices like yoga and meditation. This holistic approach recognizes the importance of treating the body, mind, and spirit as interconnected systems. More healthcare professionals are incorporating natural healing practices alongside traditional medicine to provide patients with comprehensive care.

3. Personalized Herbal Medicine: Advances in technology and personalized medicine are allowing for more customized approaches to herbal healing. With the rise

of genetic testing, healthcare providers can now offer more tailored herbal remedies based on an individual's genetic makeup, health conditions, and lifestyle factors. This approach increases the effectiveness of herbal treatments and ensures that each patient receives remedies that are best suited for their unique needs.

How to Stay Informed on New Herbal Remedies and Healing Practices

As herbal medicine and natural healing continue to evolve, it's essential to stay informed about the latest research, remedies, and practices. Here are a few ways to keep up with new developments:

1.	Read Peer-Reviewed Journals: Scientific journals focused on herbal medicine, alternative therapies, and integrative health are an excellent source of the latest research and breakthroughs in the field.

2. Follow Trusted Herbalists and Practitioners: Many experienced herbalists and practitioners share valuable insights, new trends, and educational resources through blogs, social media, and online courses.

3. Attend Conferences and Workshops: Many health organizations and herbal medicine practitioners offer conferences and workshops where you can learn about new developments in the field and connect with like-minded individuals.

Building a Sustainable, Holistic Lifestyle for Long-Term Health

Creating a sustainable, holistic lifestyle that supports long-term health involves cultivating healthy habits, nourishing your body with natural foods and remedies, and integrating wellness practices into your daily routine. This lifestyle should prioritize prevention, mental well-being, and a connection to nature. By embracing a holistic approach, you can support your body's natural healing processes, prevent illness, and achieve a state of balance that fosters vitality and well-being for years to come.

Printed in Dunstable, United Kingdom